Atlas of Pediatric Surgery

- Seong-Chul Kim
- Dae-Yeon Kim
- In-Koo Kim

Department of Pediatric Surgery
University of Ulsan College of Medicine
Asan Medical Center Children's Hospital

Atlas of Pediatric Surgery

첫째판 1쇄 인쇄 | 2009년 5월 8일
첫째판 1쇄 발행 | 2009년 5월 15일

지 은 이 김성철 | 김대연 | 김인구
발 행 인 장주연
편집디자인 박미희
표지디자인 이지선
발 행 처 군자출판사
등 록 제 4-139호(1991. 6. 24)

본 사 (110-717) 서울특별시 종로구 인의동 112-1 동원회관 BD 3층
Tel. (02) 762-9194/5 Fax. (02) 764-0209
대구지점 Tel. (053) 428-2748 Fax. (053) 428-2749
광주지점 Tel. (062) 228-0252 Fax. (062) 228-0251
부산지점 Tel. (051) 893-8989 Fax. (051) 893-8986

www.koonja.co.kr

* 파본은 교환하여 드립니다.
* 검인은 저자와의 합의 하에 생략합니다.

ISBN 978-89-6278-122-9

정가 50,000원

서문

책을 출판하는 일은 책임이 매우 큰 일이 아닐 수 없다. 가뜩이나 넘쳐나는 정보들 때문에 정신을 차리기 바쁜 세상에 또 다른 정보를 제공하겠다는 일이기 때문이다. 또 하나 늘 생각하고 있는 일은 쓸데없는 책을 출판하지 않는 것이 귀중한 자원인 종이를 아끼는 방법이고 자연보호의 첫걸음이라는 생각이다. 그럼에도 불구하고 여기 '눈으로 배우는 소아외과' 라는 책을 내는 것은 소아외과 질환의 특수성 때문이다.

소아외과 질환의 상당히 많은 부분은 선천성 기형 때문에 발생한다. 자주 발생해서 쉽게 경험할 수 있는 병도 있지만 아주 희귀하여 3차병원에서도 자주 볼 수 없는 질환이 있다. 이제까지의 학계의 관습은 증례보고를 통해 희귀질환들을 보고하고, 어느 땐가 이들을 한데 모아 병의 특성들을 정리(collective review) 하고는 한다. 어느 특정 선천성 질환을 이해하려면 이런 종합적인 보고를 읽는 것이 가장 좋은 방법이라 하겠으나, 상당한 시간을 소요해야 한다. 이 책은 비교적 전형적인 소견을 사진이나 방사선 소견으로 소개하고 요약된 설명을 붙여, 소아외과 질환을 보다 빠르고 쉽게 이해하도록 엮은 책이다.

이 책을 엮게 된 또 다른 의미는 서울아산병원 소아외과 20년 역사를 정리하는 뜻도 있다. 한 해에 1,000례 이상의 수술과, 100례 가량의 신생아 외과수술을 하는 소아외과에서 경험한 우리나라의 증례들이다. 소아외과를 공부하는 의과대학생, 외과 전공의, 소아외과 질환의 치료에 직 · 간접적으로 깊이 관여하는 산과 의사 및 소아과 의사에게 도움이 되었으면 하는 것이 이 책을 엮은 사람들의 바람이다. 이 책을 엮는데 주도적인 역할을 한 김 성철 선생과, 현재 가장 활발히 활동하면서 도움을 준 김 대연 선생 그리고 남 소현 선생에게 깊은 감사의 말씀을 드린다. 이 책을 이용하는 모든 분들이 소아외과 질환을 이해하는데 도움이 되었으면 하는 것이 우리의 희망이고, 이런 형식의 소아외과 책이 우리나라 증례들로 처음 만들어진 것에 보람을 느낀다.

이 책의 성격상 독자층이 제한적 일 수밖에 없음에도 불구하고 선뜻 출판을 결정해 주신 군자출판사의 장 주연 사장님께 감사의 말씀을 드린다. 당연히, 1989년 개원 이후, 서울아산병원 소아외과에 와서 치료를 받아 이렇게 뜻있는 책을 엮을 수 있게 해 준 환아 및 그들의 부모님께도 깊은 감사의 말씀을 드리고 싶다.

울산대학교 의과대학 서울아산병원 소아외과 김 인 구

C o n t e n t s

목차

1 Torticollis (pseudotumor of infancy, fibromatosis colli)

1) Etiology: unknown

Birth injury, abnormal obstetric position, true neoplasm, etc

2) Fibrosis of sternocleidomastiod muscle

Firm swelling and shortening of the muscle noted at or shortly after birth

3) Clinical features

Head tilted to the affected side, and chin to the opposite (Fig. 1)

Refusal of rotation to the affected side, especially with feedings

Facial and cranial asymmetry over the ensuing years

4) Diagnostic workup

Radiography of neck and spine to rule out cervical spine abnormalities

Ultrasonography, occasionally

Careful evaluation in an older child to exclude a true neoplasm

5) Physiotherapy

Passive stretching of the muscle, repeatedly each day

By turning the chin toward the affected side, and head to the opposite

6) Surgery

Division of SCM between the middle and lower third in the case of

- More than 7 to12 months of age
- Facial hemihypoplasia
- Refractory to physiotherapy

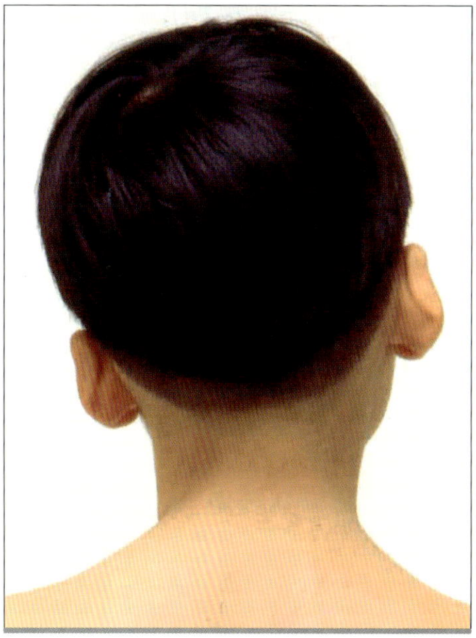

Fig. 1. Torticollis, left. The head tilted to the left side, and the chin to the right.

2 Thyroglossal Duct Cyst

1) Embryology

The thyroid is connected to the tongue at the foramen cecum during its descent by the thyroglossal duct (TGD).

This duct disappears after the completion of the thyroid descent.

The persistence of the element of the duct will result in TGD cyst.

2) Clinical features

Midline cervical cyst usually overlying the hyoid bone

Usually asymptomatic, mobile, spherical

Can be infected with oral bacteria (Fig. 2-1)

3) Diagnostic workup

Ultrasonography (Fig. 2-2)

Thyroid scanning, if ectopic thyroid suspected

4) Differential diagnosis

TGD cyst is below the strap muscle, filled with thick saliva.

Dermoid cyst

Submental lymphadenitis

Ectopic thyroid, especially lingual thyroid (cf: permanent hypothyroidism)

5) Treatment

Surgical excision of the cyst and its communicating duct to the tongue base with the central portion the hyoid (Fig. 2-3)

Incision and drainage, if infected, and delayed complete excision

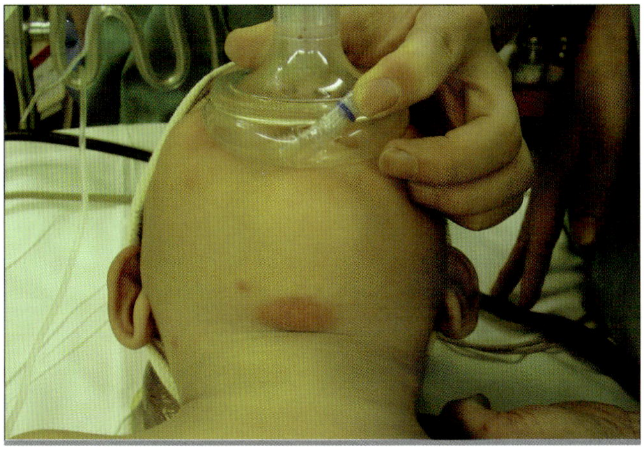

▸▸Fig. 2-1. Infected thyroglossal duct cyst.

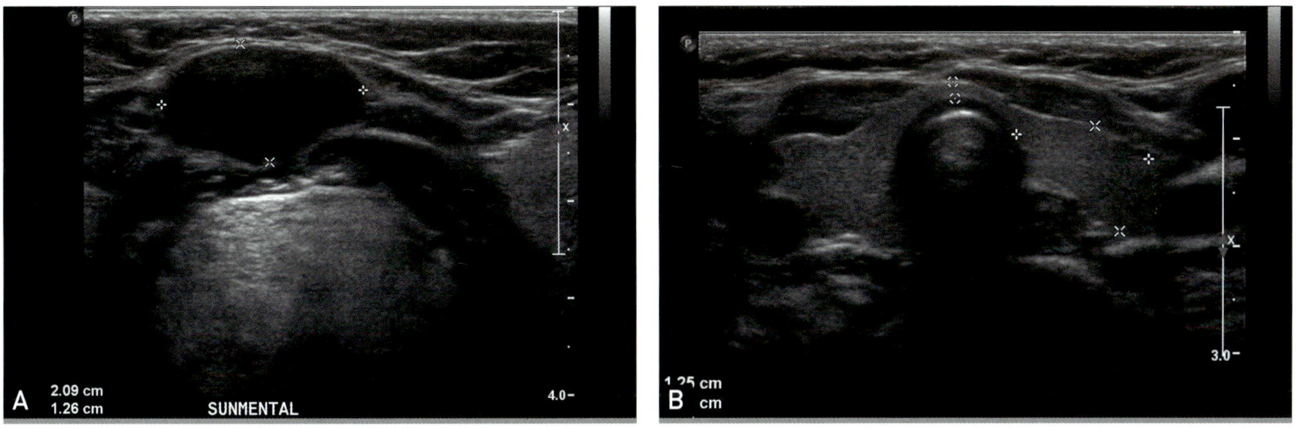

▸▸Fig. 2-2. Ultrasonograms showing submental cyst **(A)** below the strap muscles and the normal thyroid **(B)**.

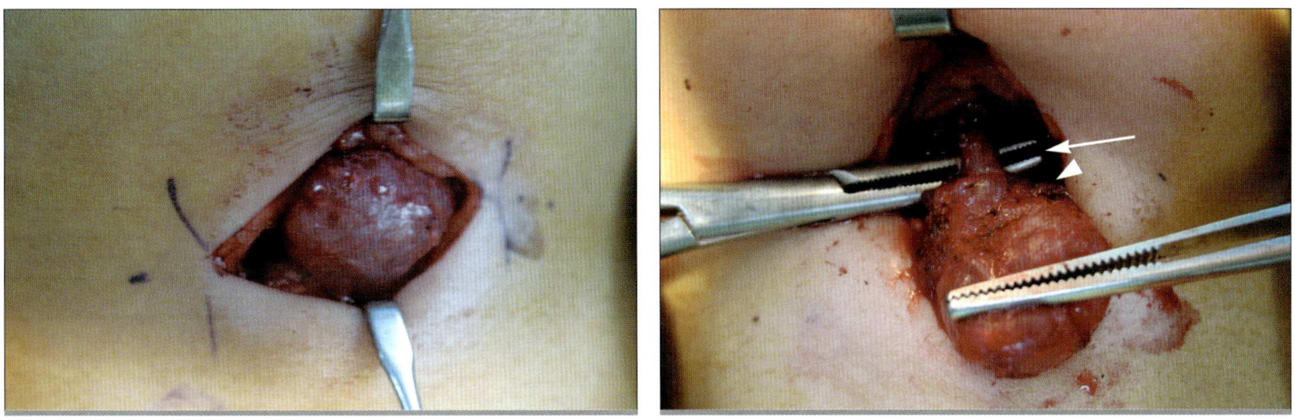

▸▸Fig. 2-3. Operative findings of thyroglossal duct cyst. Note the excised hyoid bone (arrowhead) and the duct (arrow) to the foramen cecum.

3 Branchial Cleft Anomalies

1) Incidence

2nd cleft anomaly (75%) > 1st > 3rd, 4th

2) Anatomy: Please refer to the articles for the schematic drawings.

1st anomaly:

the posterior border of the parotid → the external auditory canal

2nd anomaly:

the middle or lower third of the neck along the anterior border of the sternocleidomastoid muscle

→ over the hypoglossal and glossopharyngeal nerves

→ between the carotid artery bifurcation

→ the tonsillar fossa

Pyriform sinus fistula or cyst (3rd and 4th):

the middle or lower third of the neck along the anterior border of the sternocleidomastoid muscle

→ between the hypoglossal and glossopharyngeal nerves

→ posterior to the internal carotid artery

→ penetrate the thyrohyoid membrane

→ the pyriform sinus (3rd to the superior portion and 4th to the inferior portion)

3) Clinical features

Cyst, sinus, fistula, cartilaginous remnant

In pyriform sinus anomaly, life-threatening respiratory compromise in a neonate or thyroiditis is possible.

4) Diagnostic workup

Fistulography

Esophagography (Fig. 3-1)

Ultrasonography

Computed tomography (Fig. 3-2)

Endoscopy

5) Treatment

Surgical excision (Fig. 3-3)

Incision and drainage, if infected, and delayed complete excision

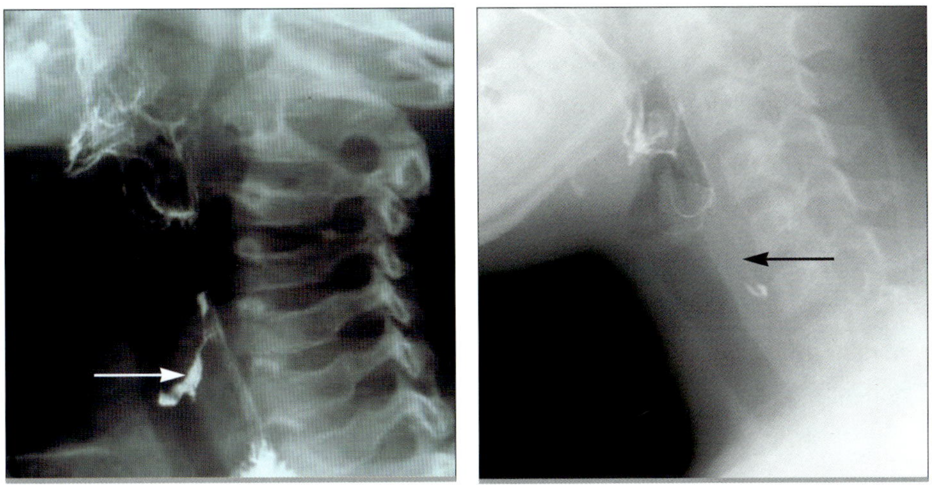

▸▸ **Fig. 3-1.** Esophagograms of pyriform sinus fistula (arrow).

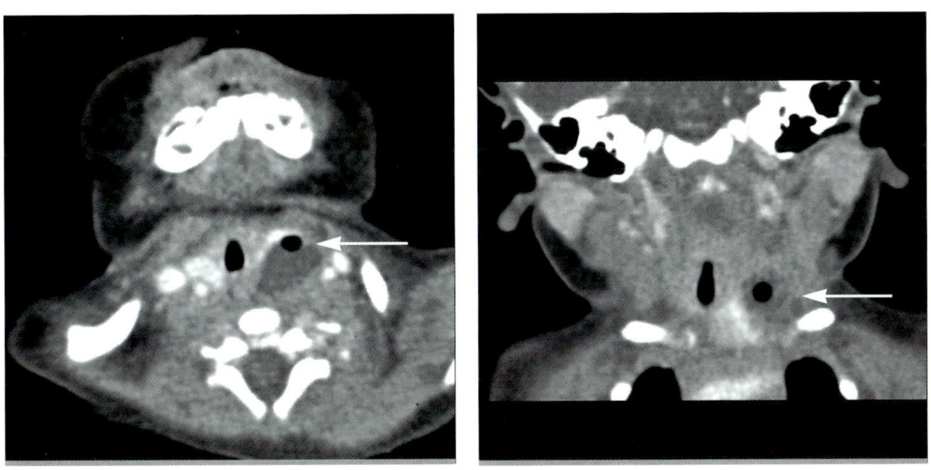

▸▸ **Fig. 3-2.** Computed tomograms of pyriform sinus cyst showing the cyst (arrow) with air bubble posterior to the thyroid.

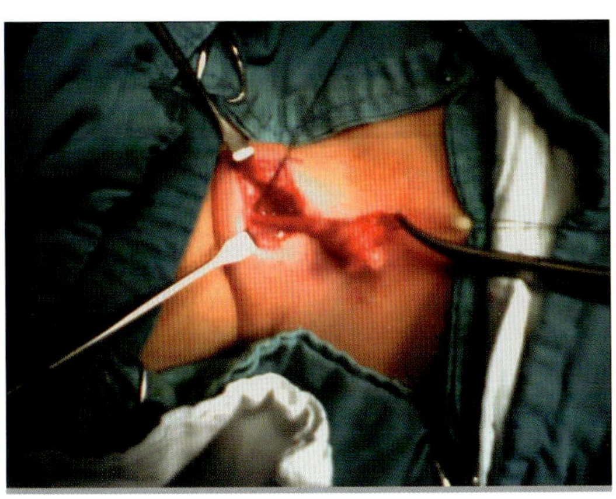

▸▸ **Fig. 3-3.** Operative finding of 2nd branchial fistula.

4 Lymphangioma

1) Classification

Infiltrative and cystic

Capillary, cavernous and cystic

2) Clinical features

More than two thirds are apparent at birth.

Appears most commonly in the neck (Fig. 4-1, 2 and 4-3)

Infection, inflammation

Sudden enlargement with internal bleeding

3) Diagnostic workup

Soft tissue density radiography

Ultrasonography

Computed tomography

Magnetic resonance imaging

4) Treatment

Surgical excision with vital structures saved (Fig. 4-3)

Sclerotherapy (Fig. 4-4) in cystic, cavernous, unresectable or recurrent case

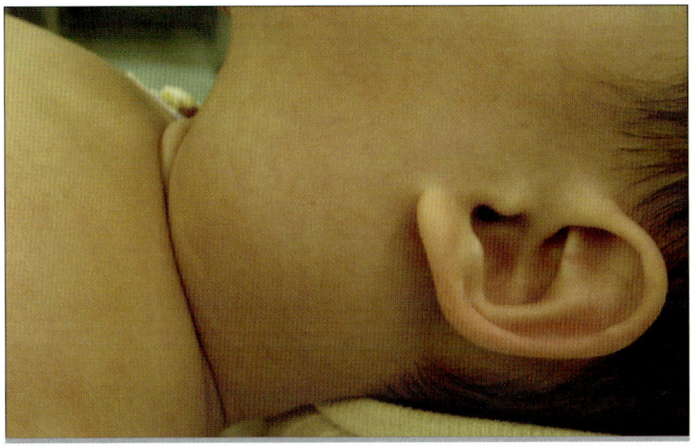

▸▸ Fig. 4-1. Small lymphangioma in the neck.

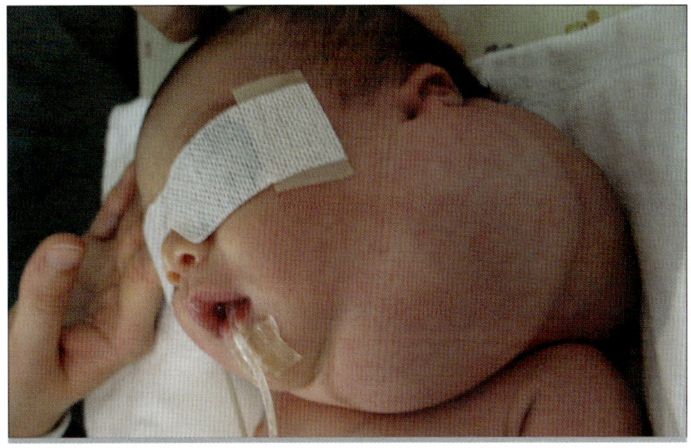

▸▸ Fig. 4-2. Huge lymphangioma in the neck with the tongue saved.

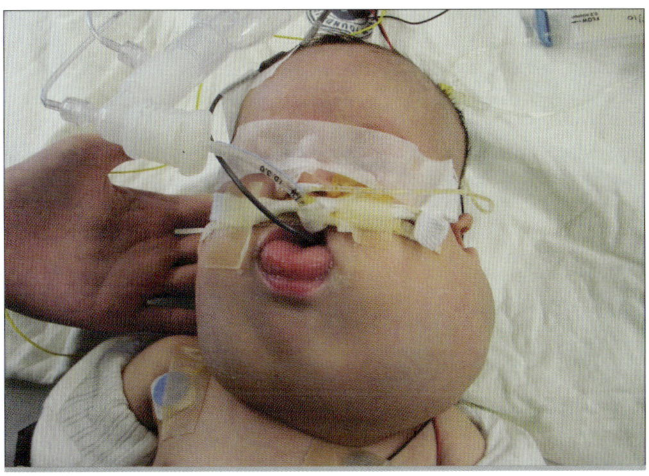

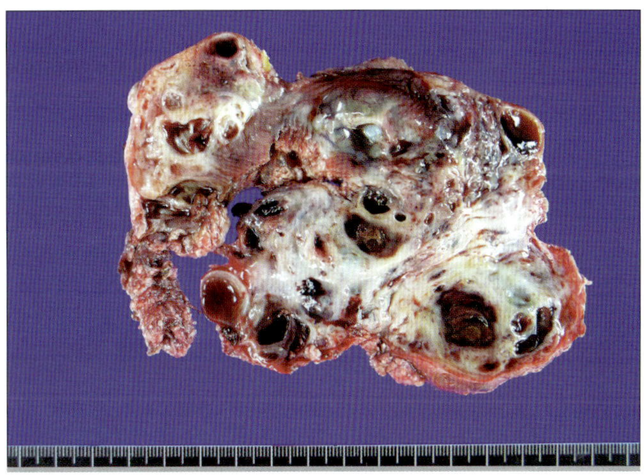

▸▸ Fig. 4-3. Huge lymphangioma in the neck with the tongue involved.

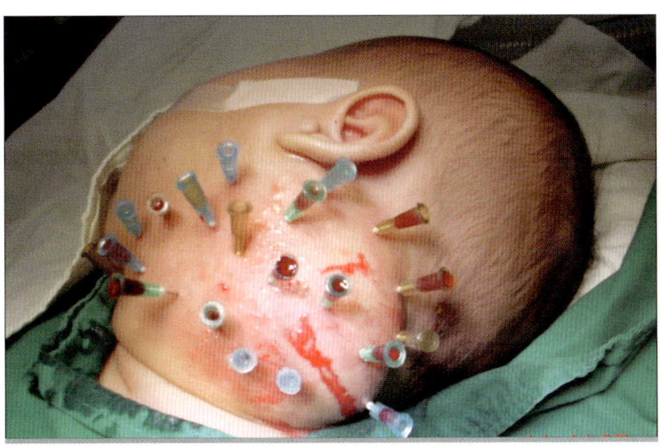

▸▸ Fig. 4-4. Sclerotherapy of lymphagioma.

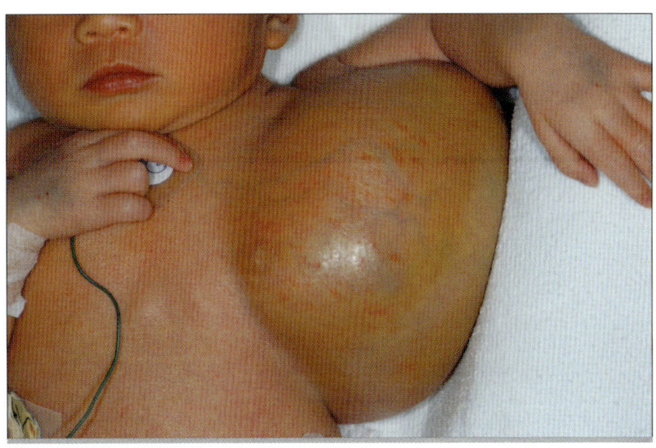

▸▸ Fig. 4-5. Lymphangioma in the axilla.

5 Esophageal Atresia (EA) and Tracheoesophageal Fistula (TEF)

1) Gross classification (Fig. 5-2)

A. pure EA without TEF (Fig. 5-3) : long gap
B. EA with proximal TEF : very rare
C. EA with distal TEF (Fig. 5-4) : the most common
D. EA with proximal and distal TEF : very rare
E. pure TEF without EA (Fig. 5-5)
F. esophageal stenosis (Fig. 5-6 and 9)

2) Clinical features

Maternal polyhydramnios
Excessive salivation (Fig. 5-1)
Choking, coughing and cyanosis on feeding
Failure to pass a nasogastric tube
Feeding possible but aspiration (+) in pure TEF without EA (Fig. 5-2 and 5)

3) Diagnostic workup

Chest radiography with a tube as far as possible in the esophagus
- The tube coiled: EA (+)
  - GI tract gas (+) : distal TEF (+) (Fig. 5-2 and 4)
  - GI gas (-) : distal TEF (-) (Fig. 5-2 and 3)

Esophagography and bronchoscopy for pure TEF
- The fistula runs downward from the trachea to the esophagus in pure TEF ("N" or "H" configuration) (Fig. 5-5).

4) Associated anomalies: VATER or VACTERL cluster

V: vertebral - spine radiography (Fig. 5-7)
A: anal - perineal inspection (Chapter 23)
C: cardiac - echocardiography
T: tracheal
E: esophageal
R: renal - ultrasonography
L: limb - inspection (Fig. 5-8)

5) Preoperative treatment

Suction drainage of the proximal esophagus

Lowering of gastric acidity

Prompt intubation with minimal ambu bagging, if needed

Echocardiography: cardiac anomaly, the side of the aortic arch

Broad-spectrum antibiotics

6) Surgery

(1) EA with distal TEF

Rt. posterolateral extrapleural thoracotomy via the 4th intercostal space

Ligation of TEF and esophagoesophagostomy: the standard

Ligation of TEF and gastrostomy (+ esophagostomy) if the gap is long

Later reconstruction with the native esophagus or esophageal substitutes

(2) Pure EA without TEF

Esophagoesophagostomy, if possible

Gastrostomy (+ esophagostomy) first and later reconstruction

(3) Pure TEF without EA

Bronchoscopic placement of a guide-wire or Fogarty catheter through the fistula

Fistula division through the lower cervical incision: right or left

Note: Many articles recommend the right approach. But, the esophagus bulges to the left of the trachea, but not to the right in the lower cervical region.

7) Complications

Anastomotic leakage and stricture (Fig. 5-9)

Recurrent fistula

Gastroesophageal reflux

Tracheomalacia: a complication of EA itself, not of the repair

8) Prognostic factors

Associated anomaly: most important

Birth weight

Pneumonia

Esophageal Atresia (EA) and Tracheoesophageal Fistula (TEF)

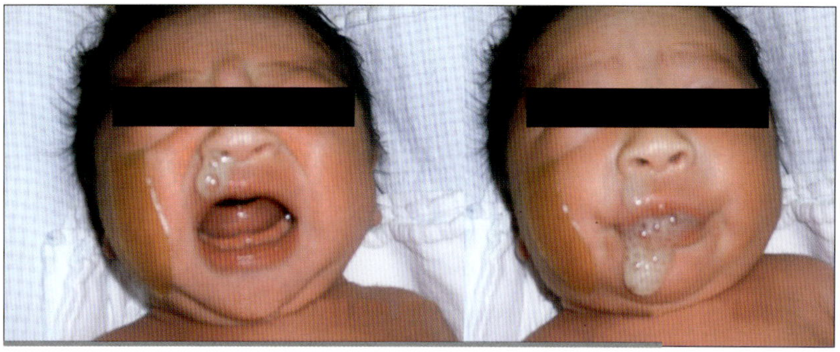

▸▸ **Fig. 5-1.** EA. Excessive salivation from the mouth and the nostril (provided by SY Chung, Chonnam National University).

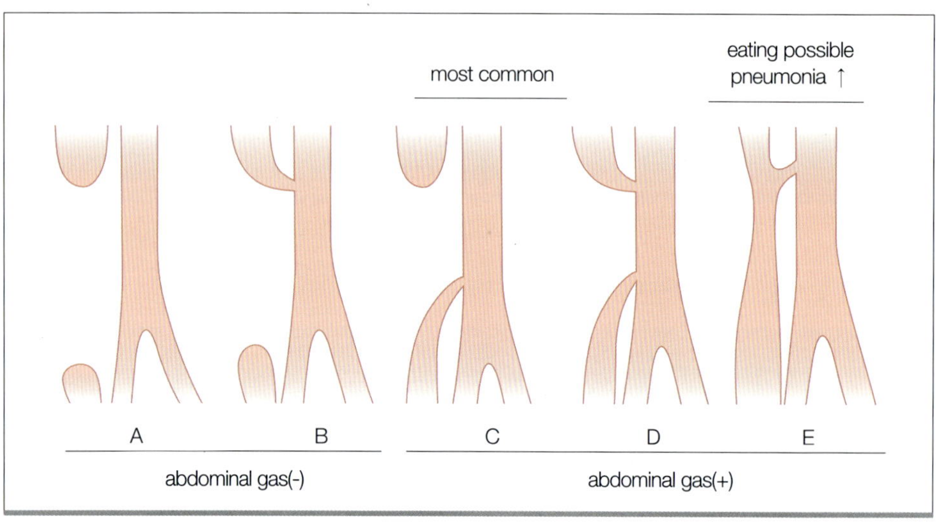

▸▸ **Fig. 5-2.** Gross classification of esophageal atresia. **A**, Pure EA without TEF. This type is usually associated with a long gap. **B**, EA with proximal TEF. **C**, EA with distal TEF, the most common of esophageal anomaly. **D**, EA with proximal and distal TEF. **E**, Pure TEF without EA. This type may be missed in the newborn period because swallowing is possible. It is associated with recurrent pneumonia.

Esophageal Atresia (EA) and Tracheoesophageal Fistula (TEF)

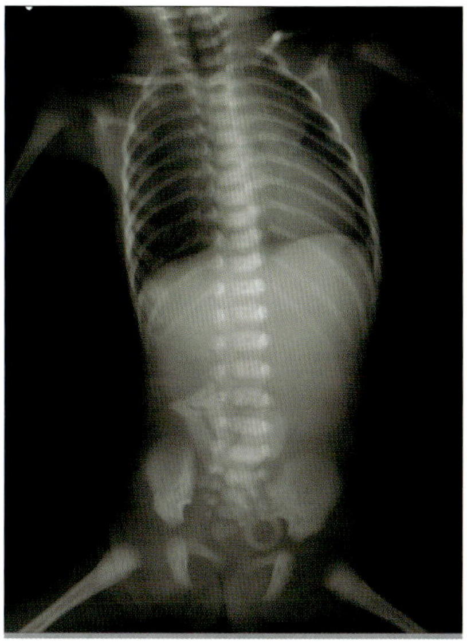

▸▸ **Fig. 5-3.** Pure EA without TEF. Plain radiograph showing the coiled nasogastric tube in the upper dilated blind pouch but no gastrointestinal gas.

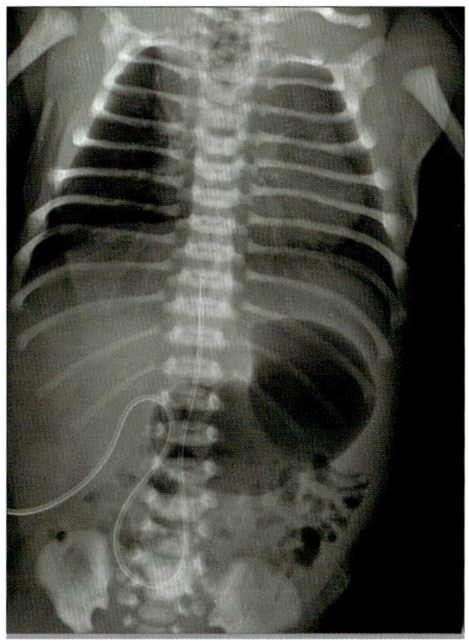

▸▸ **Fig. 5-4.** EA with distal TEF. Plain radiograph showing the coiled nasogastric tube in the upper dilated blind pouch and gastrointestinal gas.

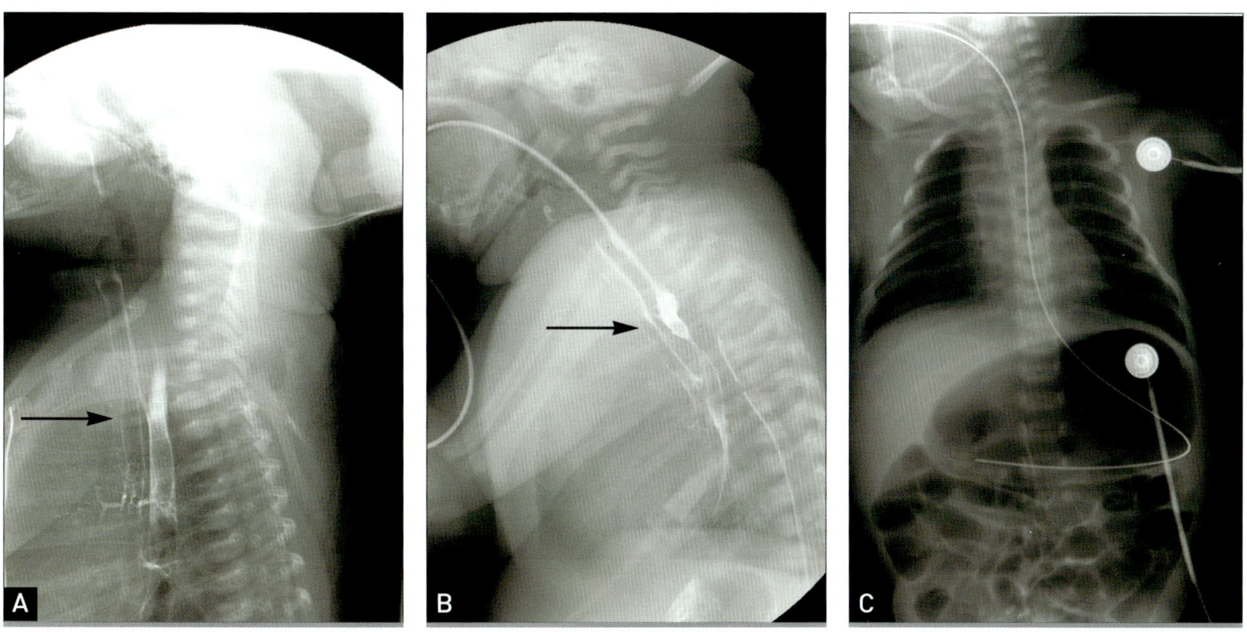

▸▸ **Fig. 5-5.** Pure TEF without EA. **A** and **B**, H or N-type TEF (arrow) is demonstrated with contrast. The upper airway is visualized with contrast through the fistula from the esophagus. **C**, A guide-wire is placed through the fistula into the esophagus under bronchoscopy, which helps to identify the fistula more easily during the operation.

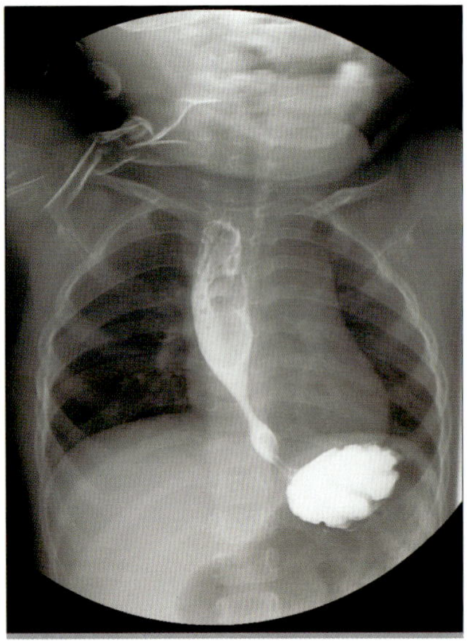

▸▸Fig. 5-6. Distal esophageal stenosis.

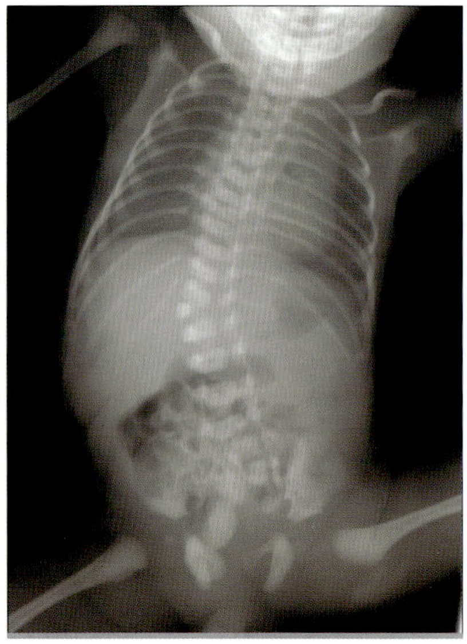

▸▸Fig. 5-7. Hemivertebra.

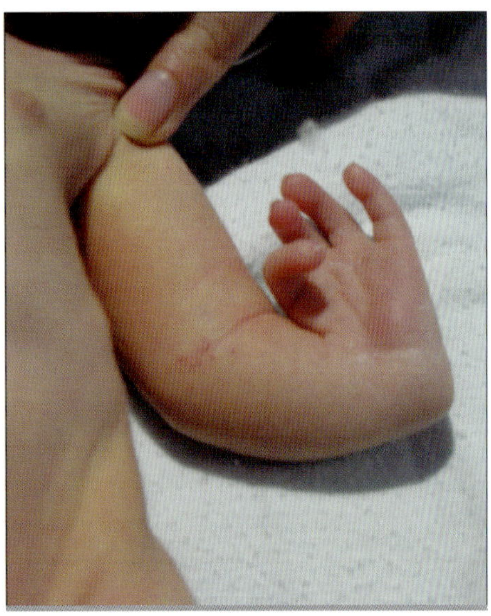

▸▸Fig. 5-8. Radial limb deformity.

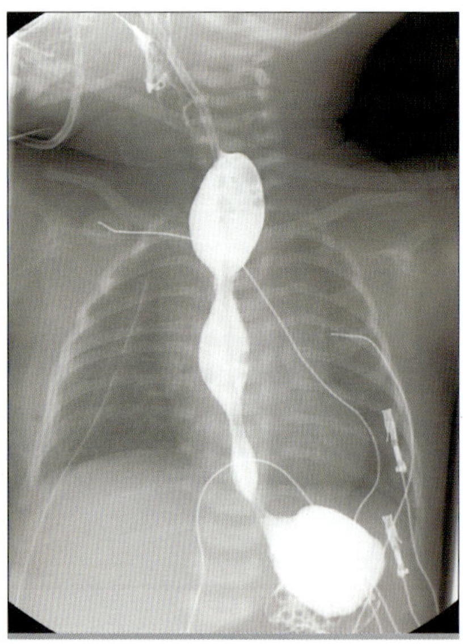

▸▸Fig. 5-9. Esophagogram 7 days after the repair of EA with distal TEF showing anastomotic stricture without leakage and distal esophageal stenosis.

6 Congenital Posterolateral Diaphragmatic Hernia (CDH)

1) Embryology

(1) Diaphragmatic anlage

The anterior central tendon from the transverse septum

The posterolateral portions from the pleuroperitoneal membranes

The dorsal crua from the esophageal mesentery

The muscular portion from the thoracic intercostal muscles

(2) Pleuroperitoneal foramen

The last area for fusion of the central and peripheral portions

Normally close during the 8th week of gestation

(3) Failure of the fusion is the cause of CDH.

2) Pathophysiology

(1) Pulmonary hypoplasia

Pressure effect by the herniated, distended bowel

(2) Pulmonary hypertension

Decrease in the number and the diameter of the arterioles

Hypertrophy of the media of the arterioles

Sensitive to hypoxia, acidosis, hypercarbia and hypocarbia

(3) Persistent fetal circulation and R-to-L shunting

Through the patent ductus arteriosus and the patent foramen ovale

3) Clinical features

Left (80%) > Right (20%) - The right diaphragm closes before the left.

Hernia sac (-) in 90%

Respiratory distress

Scaphoid abdomen

Diminished breath sounds on the side of hernia

Shift of heart sounds to the contralateral chest

Audible bowel sounds in the chest

4) Diagnostic workup

Antenatal ultrasonography

Plain chest: should include the costophrenic angles (Fig. 6-1, 2, and 6-3)

Loops of air-filled intestine within the thoracic cavity

Mediastinal shift to the contralateral side

The stomach possibly in the thorax if nasogastric tube is placed

Echocardiography

The functional status of the heart and pulmonary hypertension

Associated anomalies

5) Associated anomalies

Cardiac anomalies: the most common in the live births

Neural tube defect: the most common in the stillborn babies

Intestinal malrotation: in almost all babies

6) Prenatal treatment

Fetal karyotyping

The fetus and mother should be referred to the appropriate center.

Spontaneous vaginal delivery as close as possible to term is recommended.

Fetal intervention did not show any survival benefits.

7) Preoperative treatment: stabilization of the baby with minimal iatrogenic injury

Gastrointestinal decompression

Ventilatory support with prompt endotracheal intubation

Avoid barotrauma and oxygen toxicity (Fig. 6-4)

Minimal support with permissive hypercarbia

Two pulse oximeters for estimating R-to-L shunt

One on the right arm (preductal), the other on the lower leg (postductal)

Nitric oxide to improve pulmonary artery hypertension

High-frequency ventilation

Extracorporeal membrane oxygenation (ECMO)

Congenital Posterolateral Diaphragmatic Hernia (CDH)

8) Surgery (Fig. 6-5 and 6)

The CDH is a physiologic emergency and not a surgical emergency.

Transabdominal or transthoracic approach

Repair of the defect directly, or with a muscular flap or a synthetic patch

Tube thoracostomy, only if there is an active air leak or bleeding

- Even a small degree of negative suction may add to the barotrauma and pulmonary hypertension.

Creation of ventral hernia if necessary

9) Prognosis

Stillborn in one third

The earlier onset of symptoms, the worse prognosis.

Survival rate: 80 to 90%

10) Others forms of diaphragmatic hernia

Hiatal hernia (Fig. 6-7 and 8)

Retrosternal hernia of Morgagni (Fig. 6-9)

Diaphragmatic eventration (Fig. 6-10)

Pentalogy of Cantrell

- Anterior defect in the midline of diaphragm
- Defect in the lower part of pericardium
- Midline cleft of sternum
- Congenital heart disease
- Epigastric omphalocele

Congenital Posterolateral Diaphragmatic Hernia (CDH)

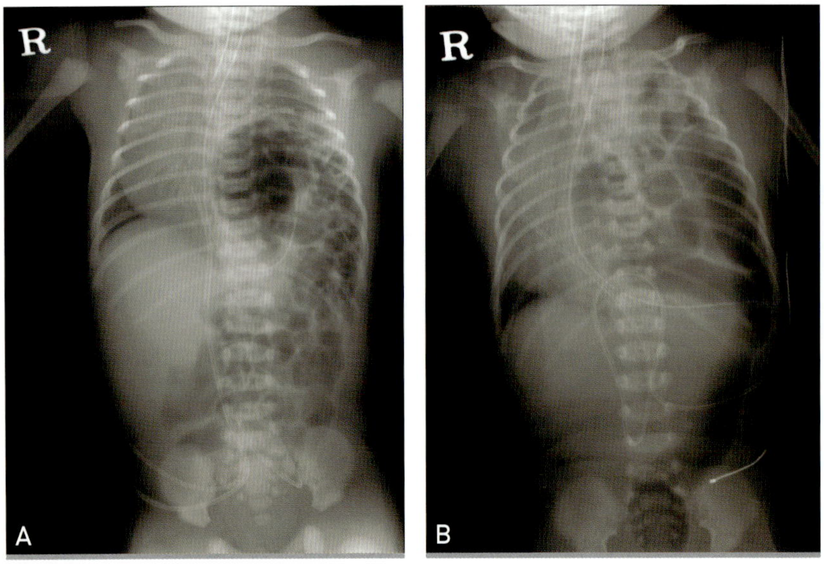

▸▸ Fig. 6-1. CDH, left. Air-filled intestinal loops in the left thoracic cavity. Also the mediastinum is shifted to the right. **A**, The stomach with a nasogastric tube is in the thorax. **B**, The tip of a nasogastric tube in the stomach is in the abdominal cavity.

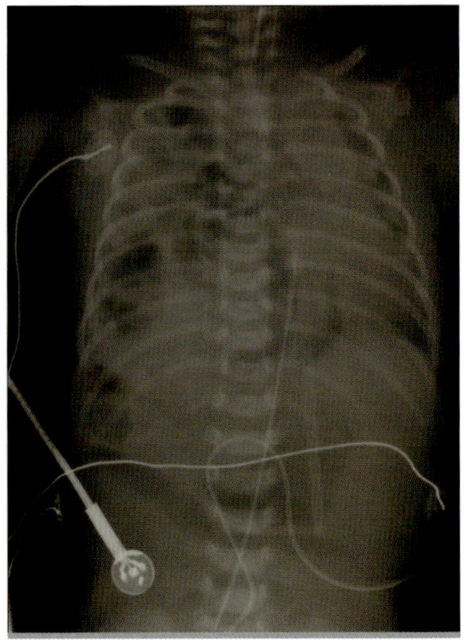

▸▸ Fig. 6-2. CDH, right.

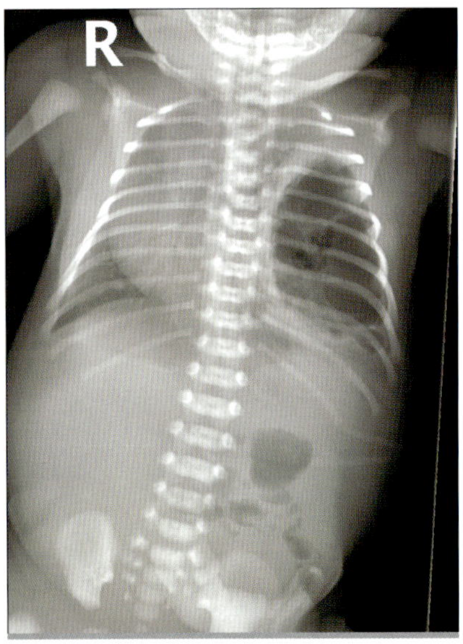

▸▸ Fig. 6-3. Congenital cystic adenomatoid malformation, left. An abnormal gas-filled cystic lesion is shown in the left thorax. But there is no continuity between the lesion and the abdominal intestine.

Congenital Posterolateral Diaphragmatic Hernia (CDH)

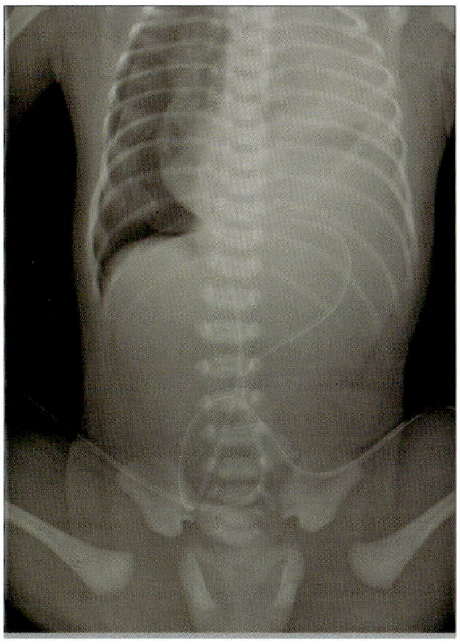

▸▸ Fig. 6-4. CDH. left. Pneumothorax in the right thorax by barotrauma. The contralateral lung is usually more vulnerable than the ipsilateral because it is more compliant.

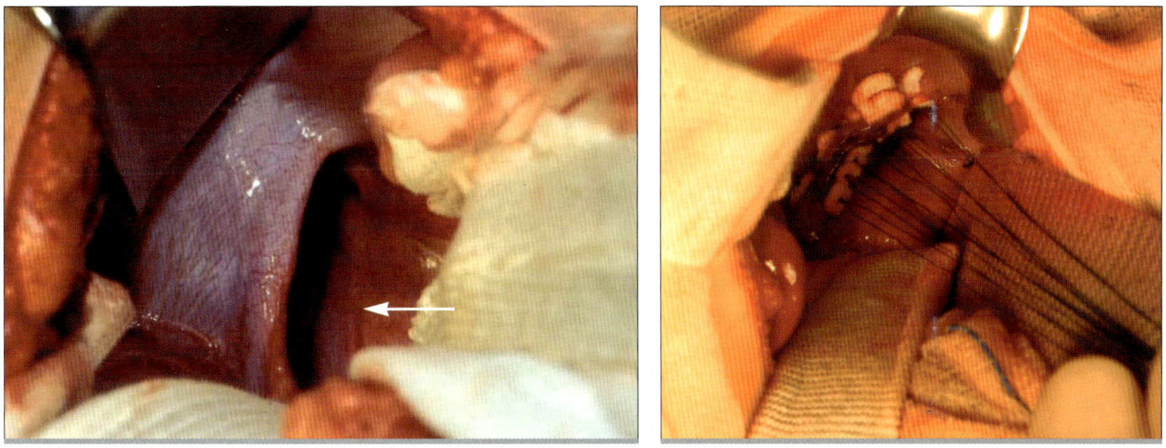

▸▸ Fig. 6-5. Operative findings of CDH. The sac is absent and the lung is not seen through the defect because of hypoplasia. The posterior rim (arrow) of the diaphragm is rolled up like a window shade by the peritoneum. The peritoneum must be opened over this fold and the diaphragmatic tissue mobilized.

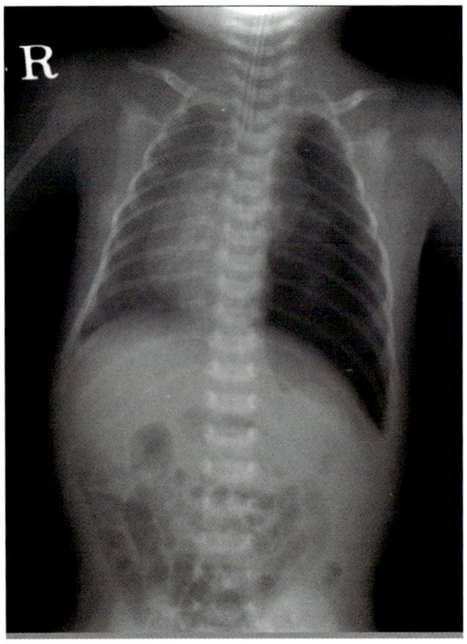

▸▸ **Fig. 6-6.** Postoperative plain film. We can see the hypopastic lung in the left thorax. Tube thoracostomy should not be done unless there is an active air leak or bleeding.

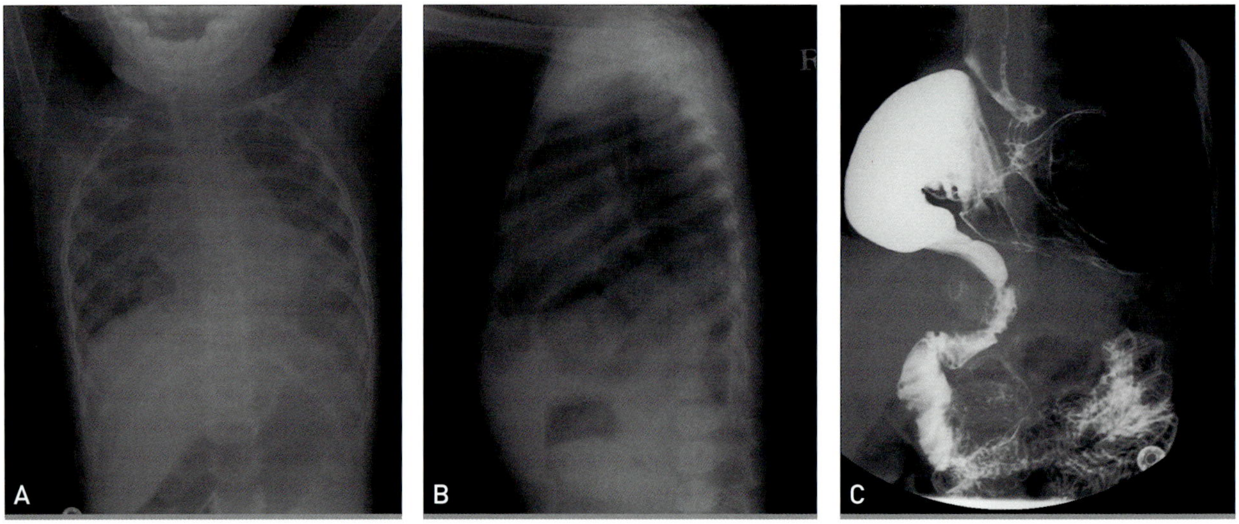

▸▸ **Fig. 6-7.** Hiatal hernia. **A** and **B**, Plain films show the herniation into the posterior mediastinum. **C**, An esophagogram shows the gastroesophageal junction and stomach in the thoracic cavity, and organoaxial volvulus of the stomach with its long axis.

Congenital Posterolateral Diaphragmatic Hernia (CDH)

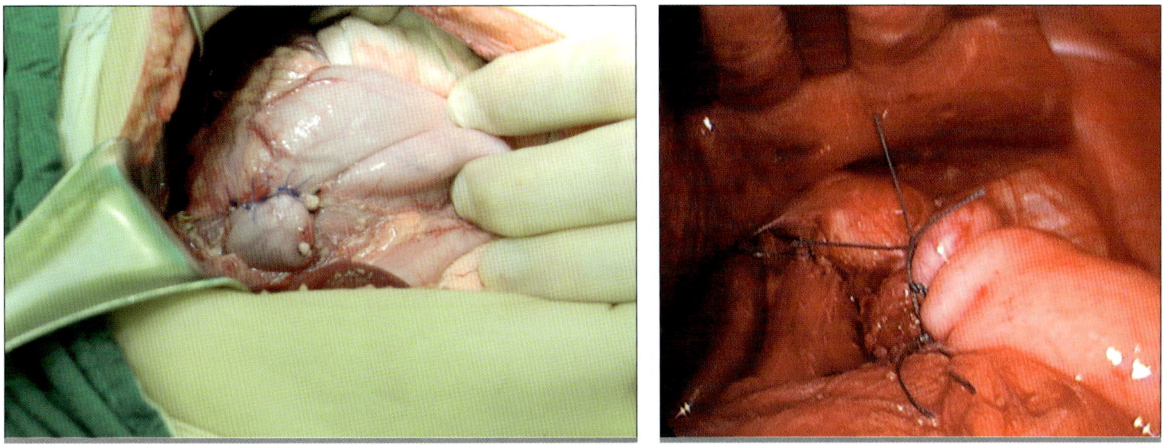

▸▸ **Fig. 6-8.** Because of the significant incidence of gastroesophageal reflux disease, fundoplication is added to the repair of hiatal hernia.

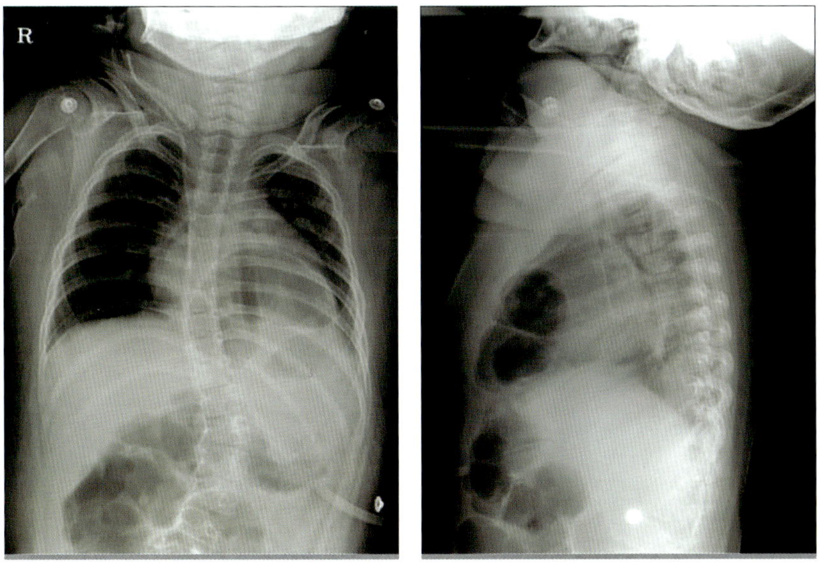

▸▸ **Fig. 6-9.** Retrosternal hernia of Morgagni. It can be located anteromedially on either side of the junction of the septum transversum and the thoracic wall.

Congenital Posterolateral Diaphragmatic Hernia (CDH)

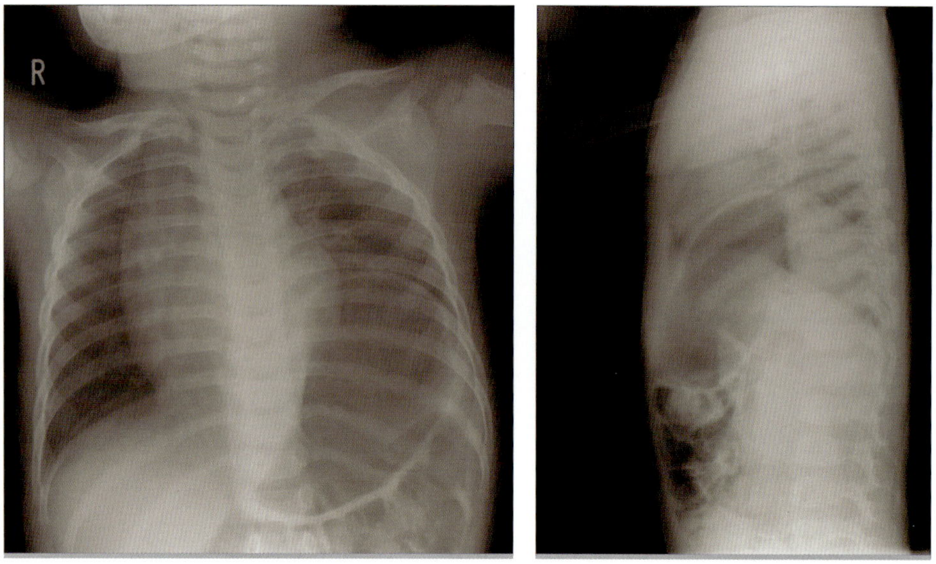

▸▸ **Fig. 6-10.** Diaphragmatic eventration, left.

7 Hypertrophic Pyloric Stenosis

1) Pathogenesis

Hypertrophy of the circular muscle fibers with no increase in numbers

The pylorus becomes thickened, edematous and stenotic.

Gastric outlet obstruction

2) Clinical features

Male to female = 4 to 1

By 3 to 5 weeks of life

Nonbilious projectile or forceful vomiting

- With high pressure induced by the hypertrophied gastric muscles

Blood (+) in the emesis, if complicated by gastritis or esophagitis

Hungry after emesis

Constipation

Dehydration and lethargy

Gastric peristaltic waves visible

Hypertrophied pyloric tumor or "olive mass" palpable

Hypokalemic, hypochloremic metabolic alkalosis

Paradoxic aciduria in severe dehydration

- Na^+ resorption with the exchange of K^+
- Na^+ resorption with the exchange of H^+, if K^+ depleted

Acid urine and hypokalemia mean that dehydration is severe.

Indirect hyperbilirubinemia: glucuronyl transferase deficiency

3) Diagnostic workup

The palpable pyloric mass is pathognomonic.

Ultrasonography (Fig. 7-1): the preferred tool

- When the olive mass cannot be palpated

Upper gastrointestinal series

4) Differential diagnosis

Feeding problem, milk intolerance

Pylorospasm, Gastroesophageal reflux

Increased intracranial pressure, metabolic disease

5) Preoperative treatment

Fluid and electrolyte balances

Nothing per os

Gastric drainage or lavage

Gastric suction during ambu bagging for induction of general anesthesia

6) Surgery

Pyloromyotomy (Fig. 7-2)

- Right upper abdominal transverse incision
- Supraumbilical curvilinear incision
- Laparoscopic

7) Complications

Incomplete pyloromyotomy

- If vomiting persists for 7 to 10 days postoperatively

Duodenal perforation

- Simple transverse closure with omental covering

Hypertrophic Pyloric Stenosis

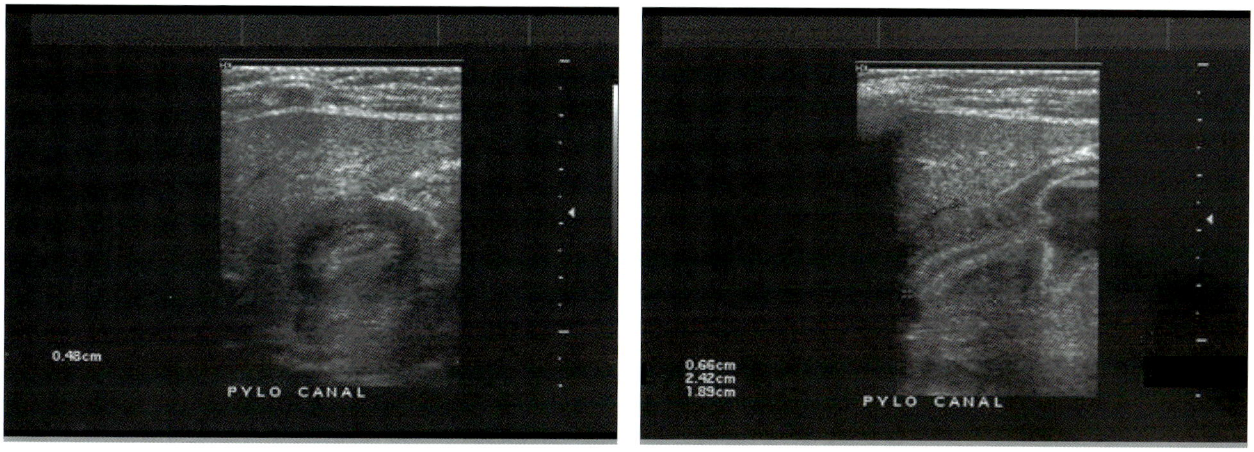

▸▸Fig. 7-1. Ultrasound images of the hypertrophied pylorus.

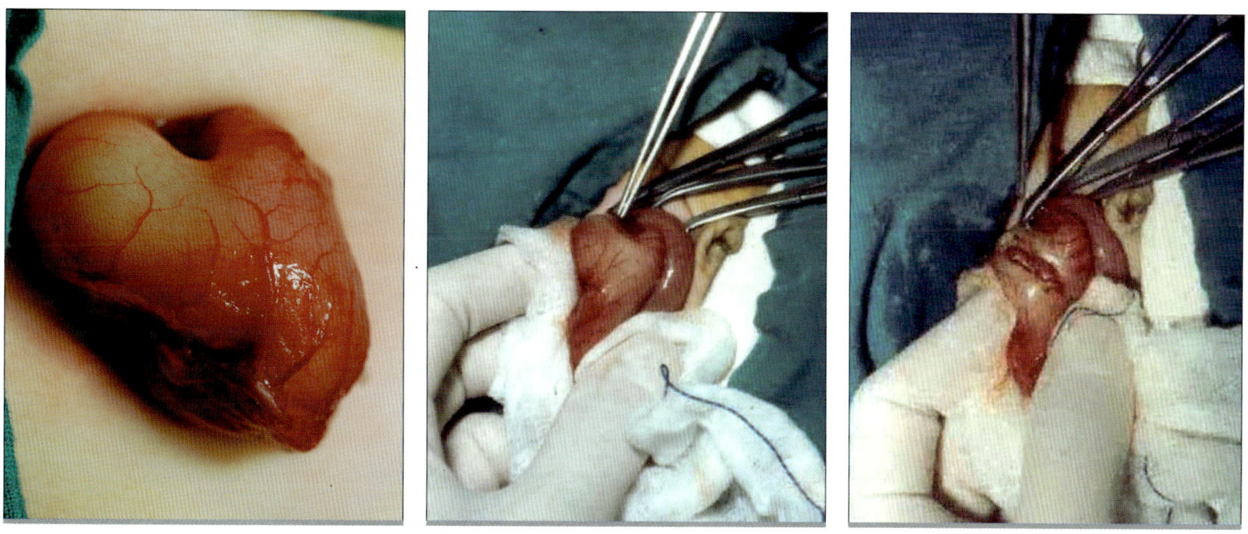

▸▸Fig. 7-2. Operative findings of hypertrophic pyloric stenosis.

8 Gastric Volvulus

1) Embryology

Lack of gastric fixation

2) Classification

Organoaxial (Fig. 6-7C): more common

Mesenterioaxial (Fig. 8-1)

3) Clinical features

Crying, colic, nausea, vomiting

Acute form : mainly in less than 6 months of life

Chronic form : mainly in adults, often in association with hiatal hernia

4) Diagnostic workup

Plain abdominal films

Upper gastrointestinal series

5) Treatment

Gastric decompression with a nasogastric tube

Gastropexy or gastrostomy

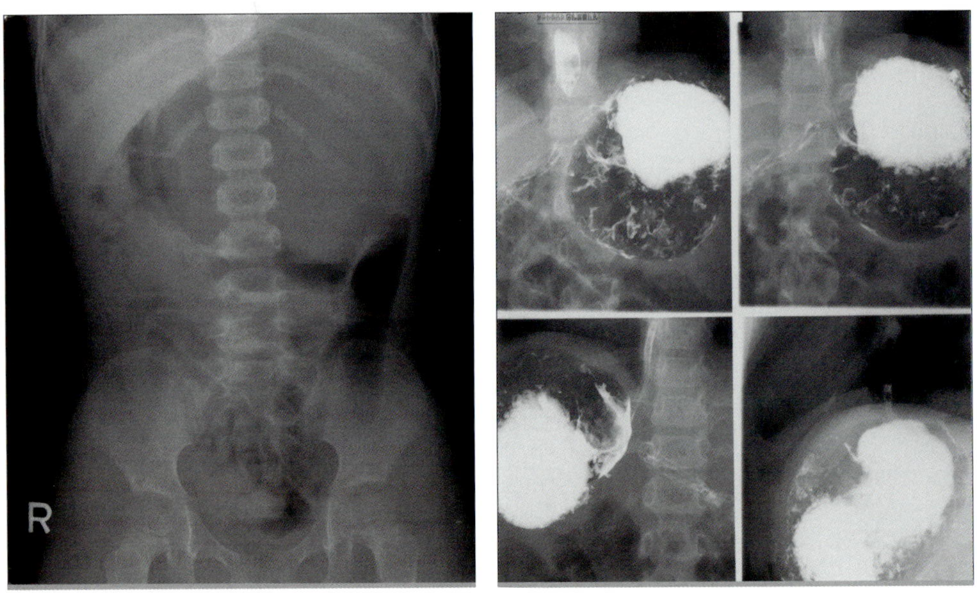

▸▸ **Fig. 8-1.** Mesenterioaxial gastric volvulus with the axis from greater to lesser curvature.

9 Midgut Volvulus

1) Embryology: Please refer to the articles for the schematic drawings.

Elongation of the intestinal tract

Physiologic herniation into the base of the umbilical cord

Return to the abdominal cavity

270° counterclockwise rotation with the axis of the superior mesenteric artery (SMA)

- Duodenojejunal loop : to the right, under and to the left of SMA
- Cecocolic loop : to the left, above and to the right of SMA

2) Normal rotation and fixation of intestine: in the first 3 months of gestation

Fixation of the duodenum at the ligament of Treitz at the left upper quadrant

Long posterior attachment of small bowel mesentery

Ileocecal valve at the right lower quadrant

Retroperitoneal fixation of the ascending and descending colon

3) Intestinal malrotation versus midgut volvulus (Fig. 9-1)

The mesenteric base becomes narrowed in malrotation, which predisposes the midgut to clockwise twisting (volvulus).

4) Clinical features

(1) Intrauterine midgut volvulus

Small bowel atresia, meconium peritonitis

(2) Acute midgut volvulus: a true emergency

30% within the first week and 50% within the first month of life

Sudden bilious emesis in a previously healthy baby

Without abdominal distension

The blood supply to the midgut from SMA can be blocked.

- Bowel strangulation will be issued.
- Midgut: from the 2nd duodenum to the distal transverse colon
- Collaterals from the celiac trunk and inferior mesenteric artery
    - The proximal and distal part of midgut will be saved.

"Midgut volvulus should be assumed in a healthy baby (esp. neonate or infant) with sudden onset of bilious vomiting until proven otherwise."

(3) Chronic midgut volvulus

More common in children older than 2 years

Midgut Volvulus

By lymphatic or venous obstruction

Chronic vomiting, intermittent colic, diarrhea, hematemesis, constipation

5) Diagnostic workup

Plain abdomen (Fig. 9-2): gasless abdomen or duodenal dilatation, but often nondiagnostic

Ultrasonography (Fig. 9-3): the preferred, whirlpool flow of SMV around SMA

Computed tomography (Fig. 9-4)

Upper gastrointestinal series (Fig. 9-5): corkscrew-like deformity of the duodenum

6) Surgery: a true emergency

Evisceration of the bowel and inspection of the mesenteric root

Detorsion of the twisted bowel in a counterclockwise direction (Fig. 9-6)

Lysis of Ladd's peritoneal band

Lysis of the anterior leaflet of the mesentery along SMA

Mesenteric widening

Appendectomy: abnormal position of the appendix

Small intestine to the right and colon to the left of the abdomen

Mesenteric fixation: unnecessary

Second look procedure: for massive strangulation (Fig. 9-7)

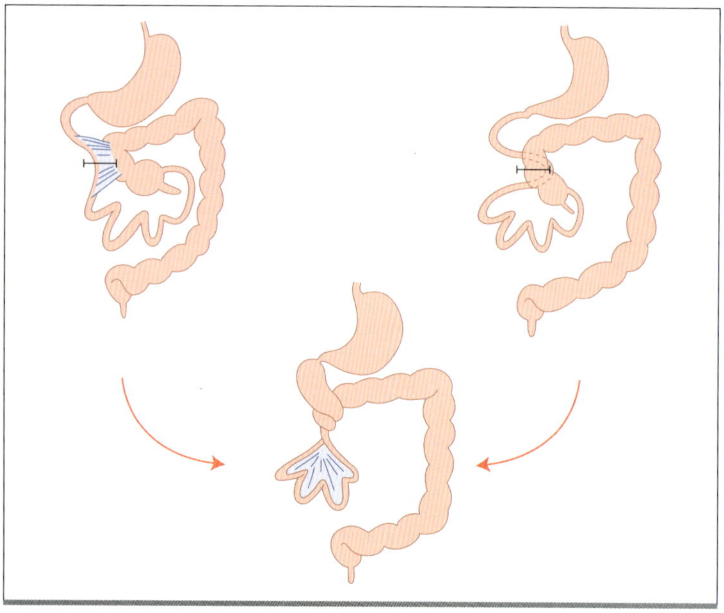

▸▸ **Fig. 9-1.** Pathophysiology of midgut volvulus. The mesenteric base is narrow in nonrotation or incomplete rotation, which predisposes the midgut to clockwise twisting.

Midgut Volvulus

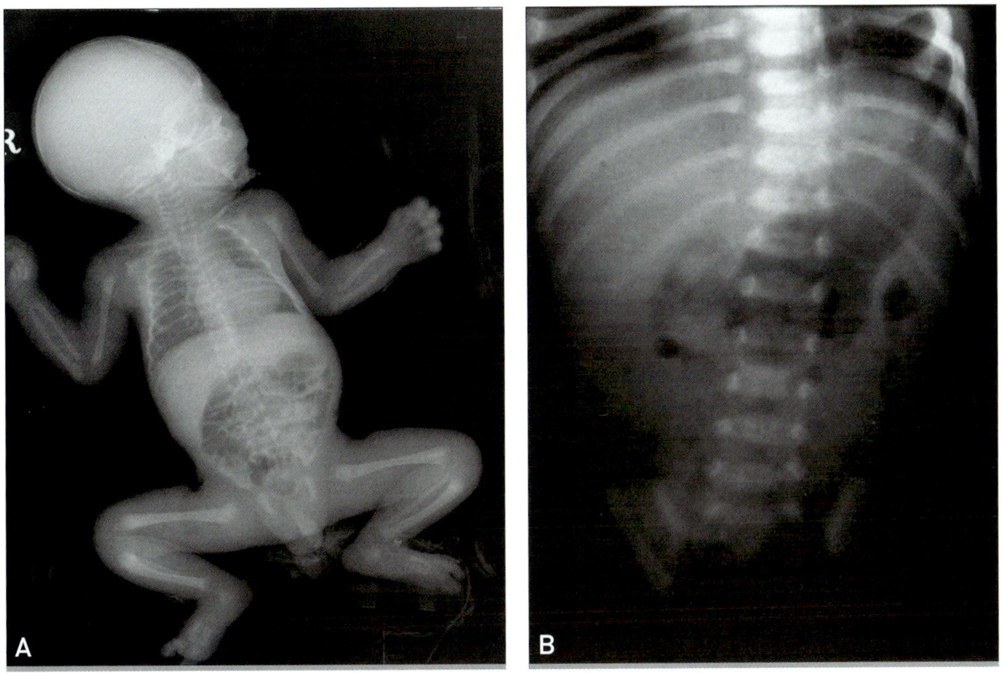

▸▸ **Fig. 9-2.** Midgut volvulus. Plain films showing nonspecific findings **(A)** and gastric distension **(B)** with the gasless distal bowel.

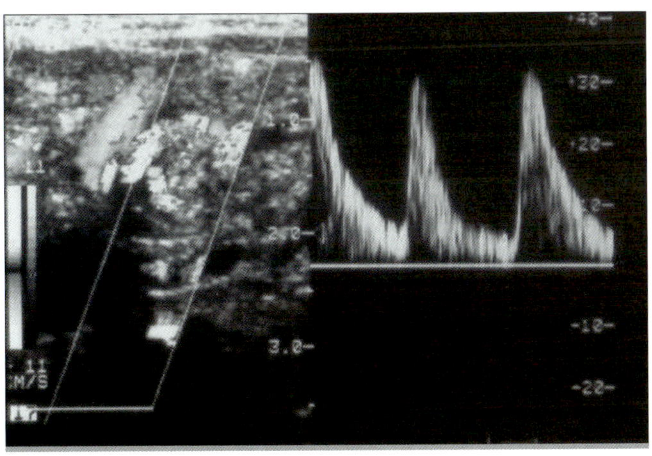

▸▸ **Fig. 9-3.** Ultrasonogram showing the whirlpool flow pattern and intact blood flow.

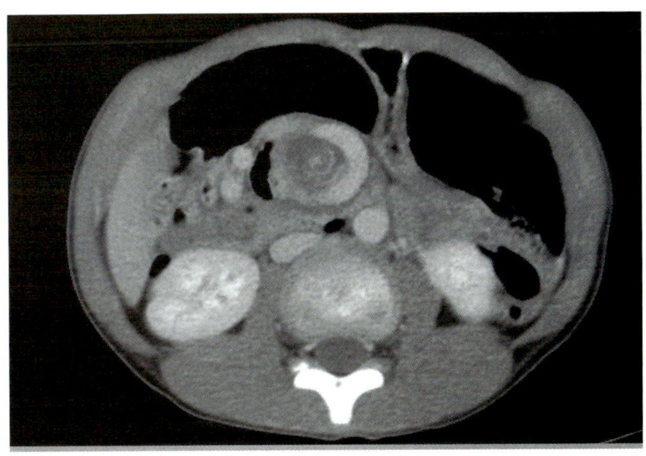

▸▸ **Fig. 9-4.** Computed tomogram showing the whirlpool flow pattern.

Midgut Volvulus

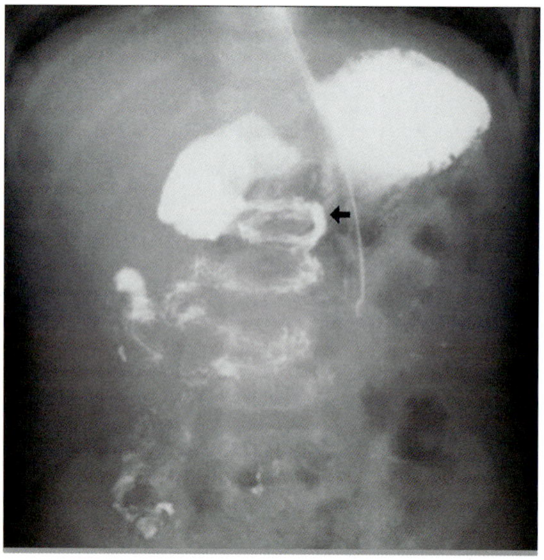

▸▸ **Fig. 9-5.** Midgut volvulus. Contrast study showing the ligament of Treitz at the midline and below the gastric outlet, and corkscrew-like deformity of the duodenum.

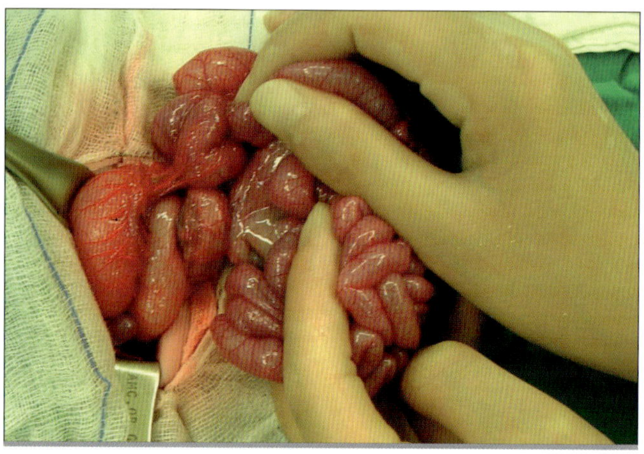

▸▸ **Fig. 9-6.** Operative findings of midgut volvulus. The whole intestine can be eviscerated from the abdominal cavity and twists in a clockwise direction. The blood supply to the intestine is intact.

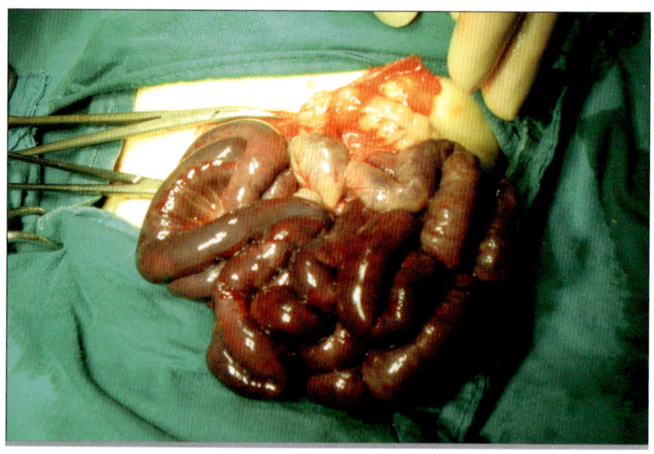

▸▸ **Fig. 9-7.** Operative findings of midgut volvulus with strangulation. There is no return of the color, peristalsis and arterial pulsation of the bowel even after detorsion.

10 Duodenal Atresia

1) Embryology

Gut tube formation from the 4th week of gestation

Obliteration of the lumen by epithelial proliferation

Vacuolization and recanalization in the 8th to 10th week of gestation

2) Etiology

The failure of recanalization

Annular pancreas

3) Clinical features (Table 10-1)

Trisomy 21 in one third

Maternal polyhydramnios in 30 to 65%

Vomiting within a few hours of birth

- Bilious (85%): duodenal obstruction distal to the ampulla of Vater
- Nonbilious (15%): obstruction proximal to the ampulla of Vater

Abdominal distension (-)

Table 10-1. Differential Diagnosis of the Proximal and Distal Bowel Obstruction

	Proximal	Distal
Vomiting	early, frequent	late
Abdominal distension	mild	severe
Dilated loops	few	many
Micro-colon	no	yes
Prostration	early	late

4) Diagnostic workup

Plain abdomen (Fig. 10-1): double bubble sign of the gas-filled stomach and 1st duodenum

Ultrasonography

Upper gastrointestinal series: in the partial duodenal obstruction

5) Surgery (Fig. 10-2)

Confirm the distal patency

Side to side duodenoduodenostomy, or web excision

Duodenal Atresia

With or without duodenoplasty or plication

Do not divide the overlying pancreatic tissue in annular pancreas

Alert windsock deformity in duodenal web with fenestration

Alert the ampulla of Vater

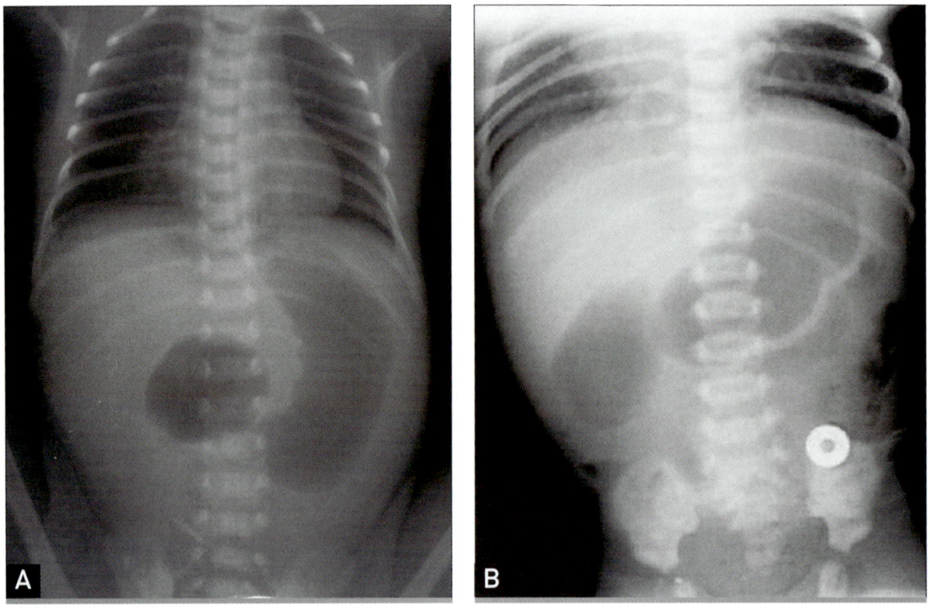

▸▸ **Fig. 10-1.** Double bubble sign. Note that Fig. **A** shows no distal gas in contrast to Fig. **B**.

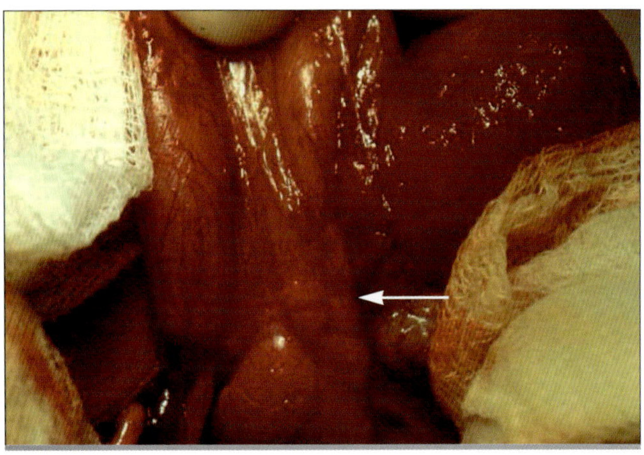

▸▸ **Fig. 10-2.** Operative findings of duodenal atresia with annular pancreas(arrow). Note prestenotic dilatation and poststenotic collapse of the duodenum.

11 Jejunoileal Atresia

1) Etiology

Intrauterine vascular insults, such as volvulus, internal hernia, or intussusception

2) Clinical features (Table 10-1)

Much lower incidence of associated anomalies than in duodenal atresia

Maternal polyhydramnios

Bilious vomiting

Abdominal distension, especially in ileal atresia

Failure to pass the meconium in the first 24 to 48 hours of life

Sometimes associated with meconium peritonitis

3) Diagnostic workup

Plain abdominal films

 Jejunal (Fig. 11-1) versus ileal (Fig. 11-2): the number of dilated loops

Contrast enema: unused microcolon in ileal atresia (Also, refer to Chapter 13)

Small bowel series in carefully selected cases with partial obstruction

4) Differential diagnosis

Meconium ileus

Total colonic aganglionosis

Colonic atresia

5) Surgery (Fig. 11-3, 4, 5 and 11-6)

Confirm the distal patency with a catheter, air or saline

Excision of atretic segment and end-to-end or end-to-back anastomosis

 With or without enteroplasty or plication

Various types of enterostomy

Bowel lengthening procedures, if short bowel syndrome anticipated

Jejunoileal Atresia

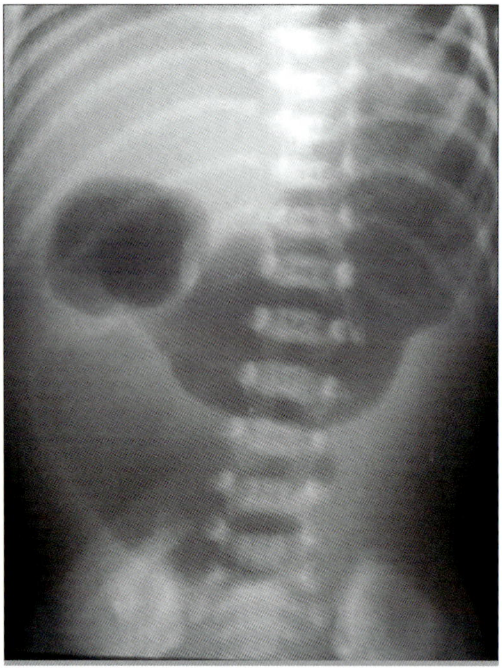

▸▸**Fig. 11-1.** Jejunal atrersia. Plain film showing the dilated stomach, duodenum and proximal jejunum.

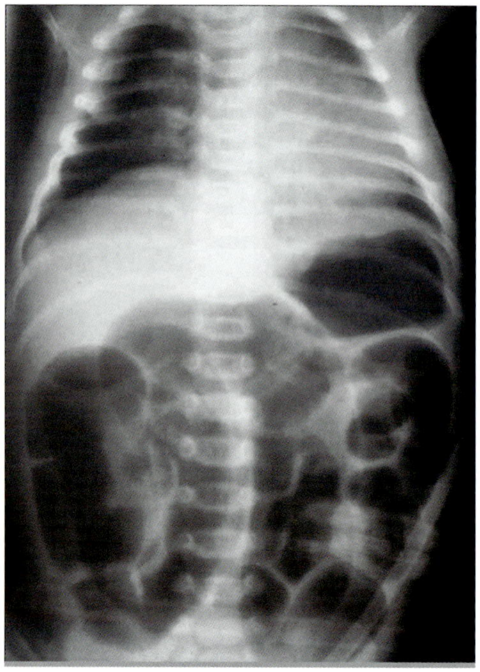

▸▸**Fig. 11-2.** Ileal atresia. Plain film showing the multiple dilated loops of intestine.

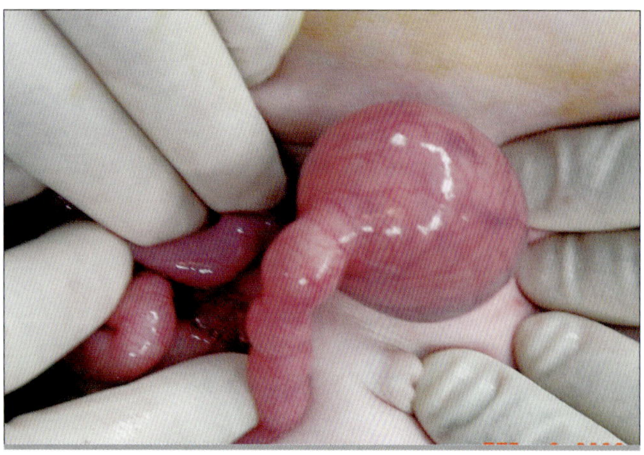

▸▸**Fig. 11-3.** Operative findings of jejunal web.

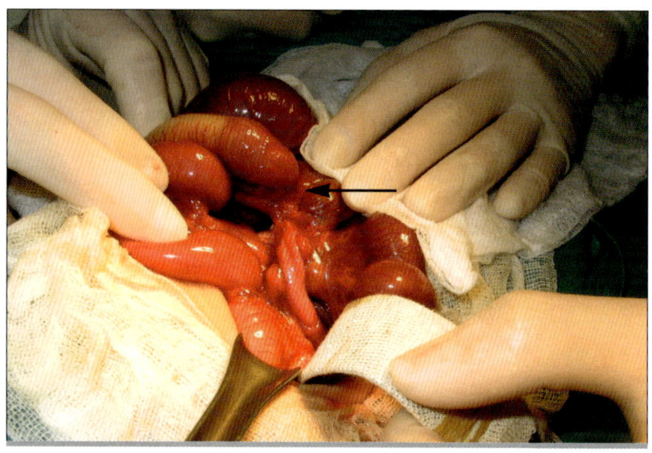

▸▸**Fig. 11-4.** Operative findings of ileal atresia (arrow).

Jejunoileal Atresia

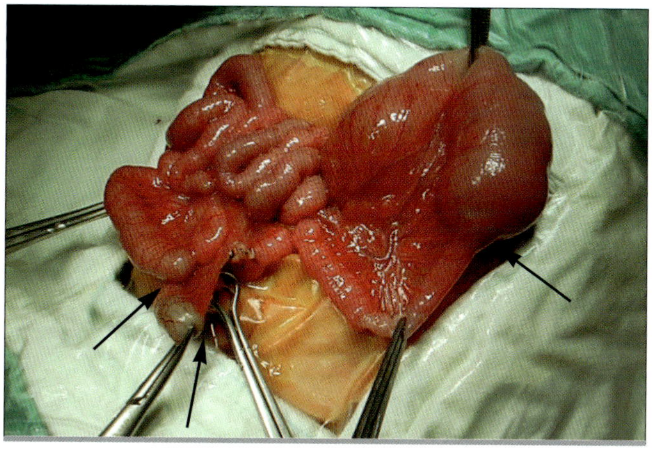

▸▸Fig. 11-5. Operative findings of multiple jejunoileal atresia (arrow).

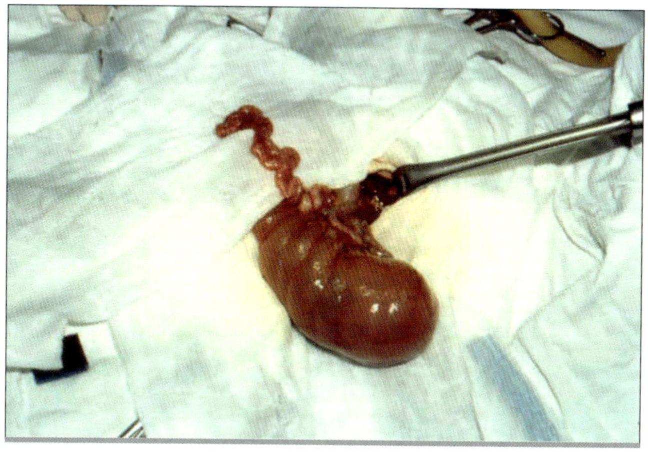

▸▸Fig. 11-6. Operative findings of apple peel or Christmas tree deformity. The distal ileum derives its entire blood supply from the ileocolic artery.

12 Meconium Peritonitis

1) Etiology

An aseptic, chemical or foreign-body peritonitis by spillage of meconium from intrauterine perforation of the intestinal tract

2) Classification

Generalized

Fibroadhesive

Cystic

Healed

3) Clinical features (Fig. 12-1)

Abdominal distension

Bilious vomiting

Cellulitis of the abdominal wall

4) Diagnostic workup

Plain abdominal radiography (Fig. 12-2, 4A, 5A and 12-5B)

- Features of intestinal obstruction
- Intra-abdominal calcifications
- Calcifications in the patent processus vaginalis or scrotum

Ultrasonography

- Pre- or postnatally

5) Surgery: evacuate the inspissated meconium in the distal bowel, if present

Resection and anastomosis (Fig. 12-3)

Enterostomy

Peritoneal drainage and the 2nd look operation (Fig. 12-4, 5 and 12-6)

- Even if there are some controversies, this procedure can save the baby by itself, or rescue the baby from an acute stage.

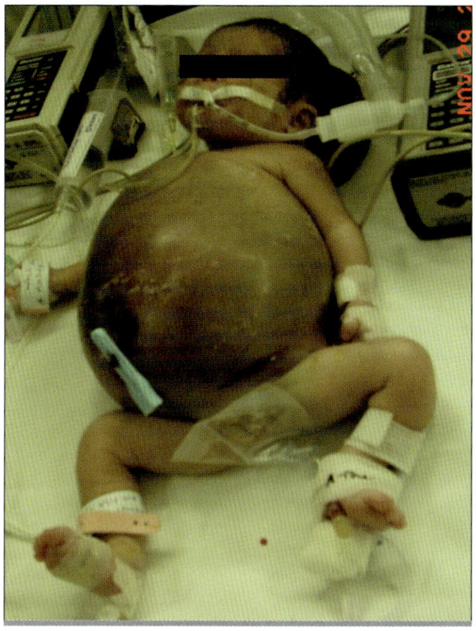

▸▸ Fig. 12-1. Meconium peritonitis. Abdominal distension, and erythema, edema and bluish discoloration of abdominal wall because of intraperitoneal meconium from intestinal perforation.

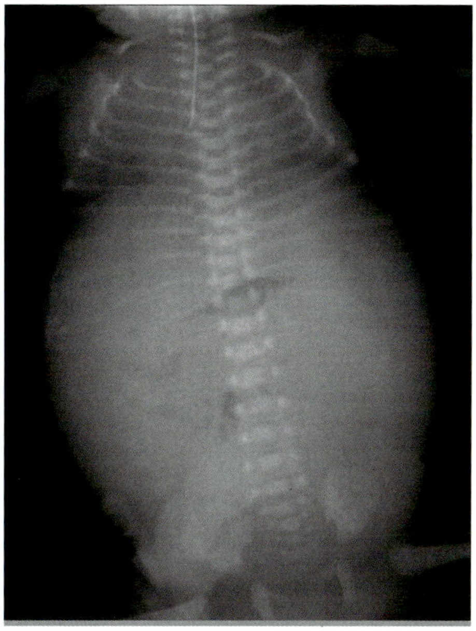

▸▸ Fig. 12-2. Plain abdominal film showing intraperitoneal calcifications on the surface of liver and abdominal distension with small amount of intestinal gas.

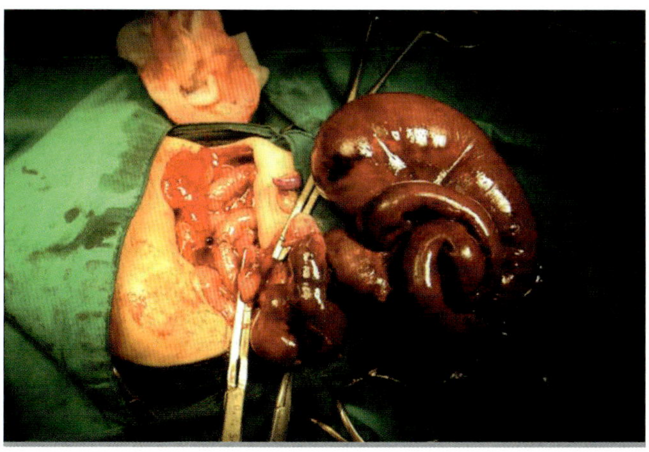

▸▸ Fig. 12-3. Operative findings showing segmental volvulus of small intestine with strangulation.

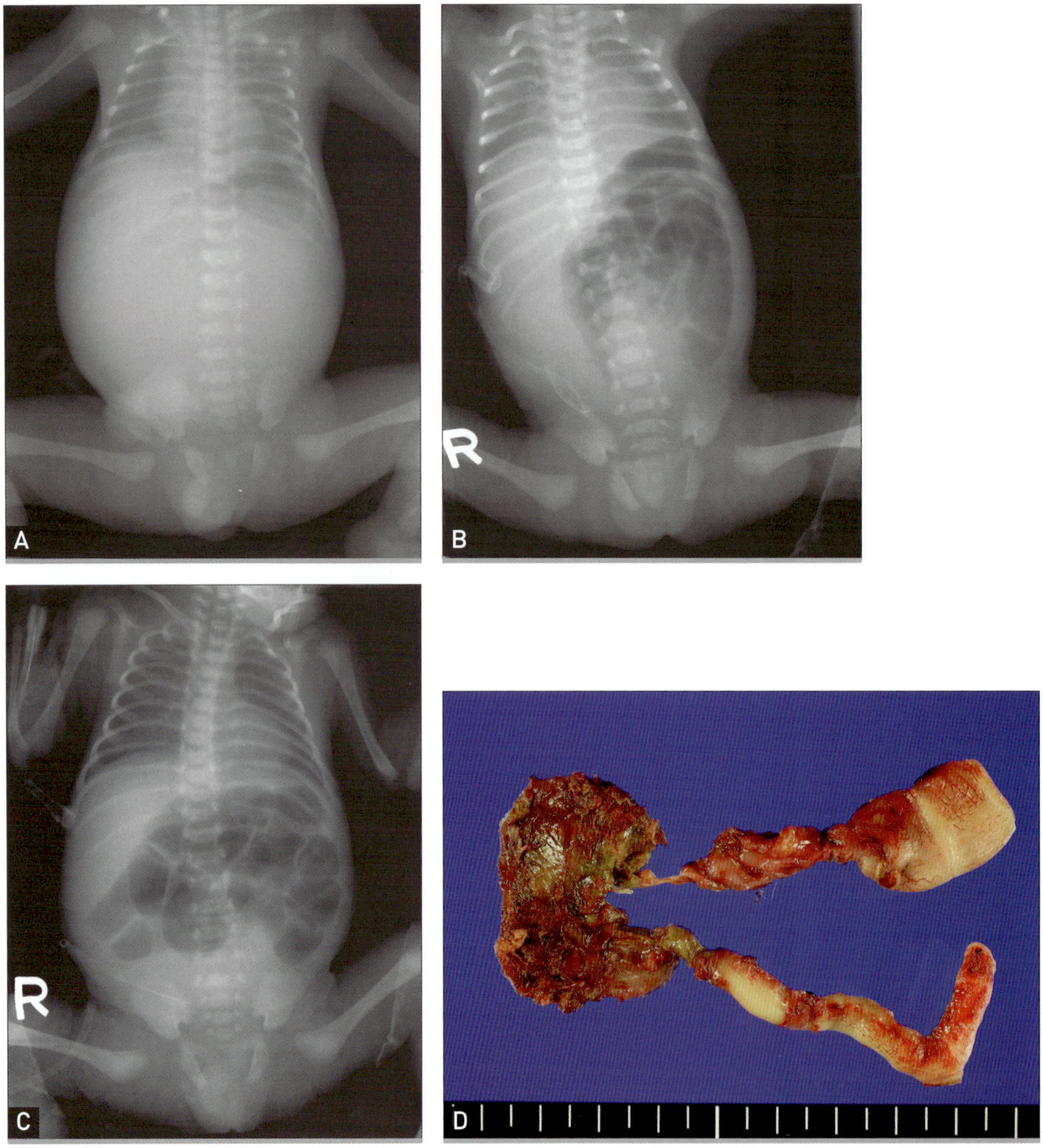

▸▸ **Fig. 12-4.** Cystic meconium peritonitis. **A**, Plain film of a newborn infant shows abdominal distension but no calcifications. The exploratory laparotomy showed a huge serous pseudocyst with severe inflammation which could not permit the entrance to the proper peritoneal cavity. Only closed suction drainage of the cyst was done. **B** and **C**, Serial follow-up films showing the progressive descent of the intestinal gas. **D**, The 2nd look operation 6 weeks of life revealed ileal atresia and a shrunken pseudocyst.

Meconium Peritonitis

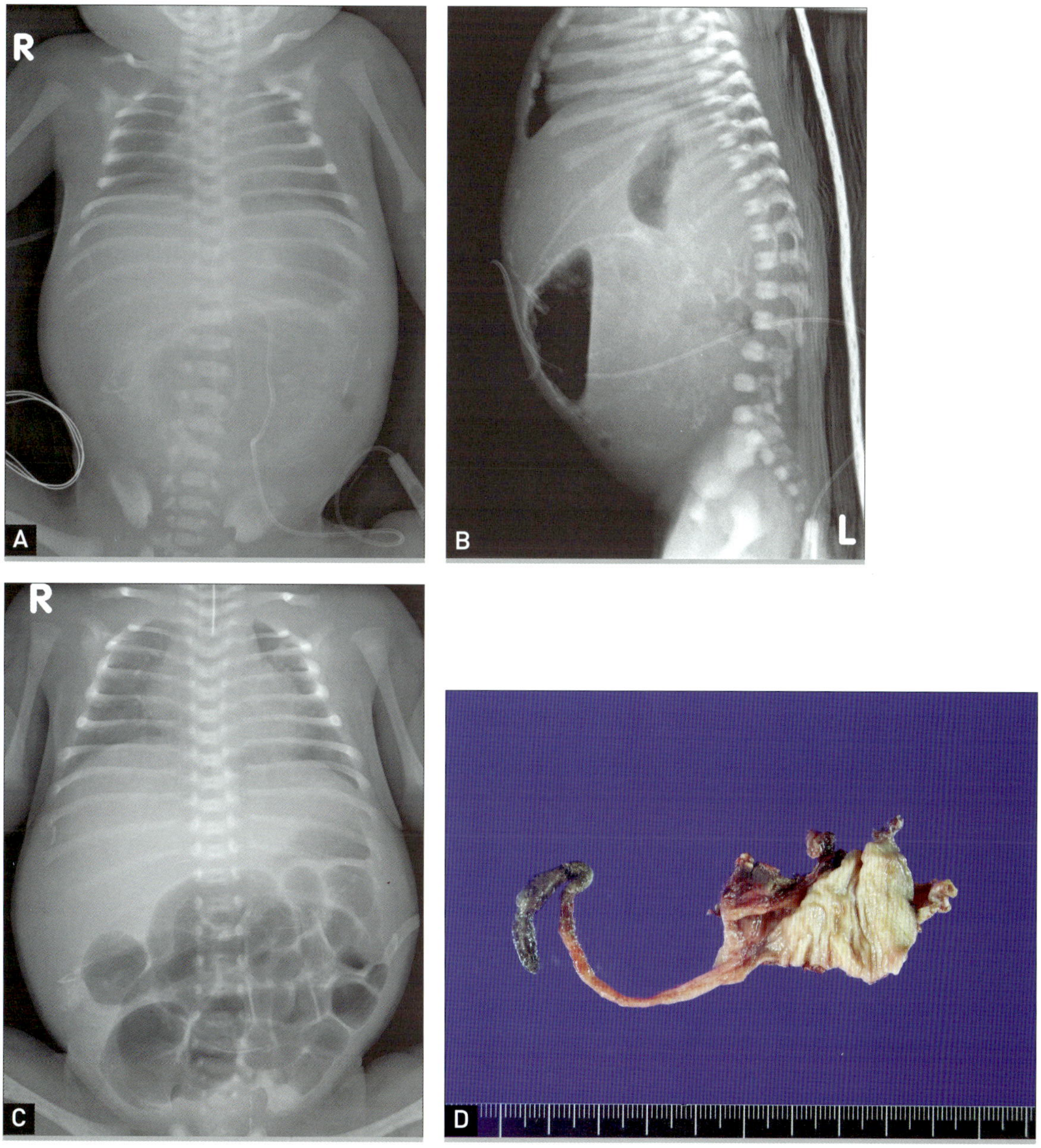

▸▸ **Fig. 12-5.** Cystic meconium peritonitis. **A** and **B**, Plain films of a newborn infant show abdominal distension with calcifications and a huge gas-filled cyst. The exploratory laparotomy showed a huge meconium-filled pseudocyst with severe inflammation. We could neither enter the proper peritoneal cavity nor find the site of meconium spillage. Only irrigation and closed suction drainage of the cyst was done. **C**, Follow-up film showing the progressive descent of the intestinal gas. **D**, The 2nd look operation 4 weeks of life revealed ileal atresia with intussusception.

Meconium Peritonitis

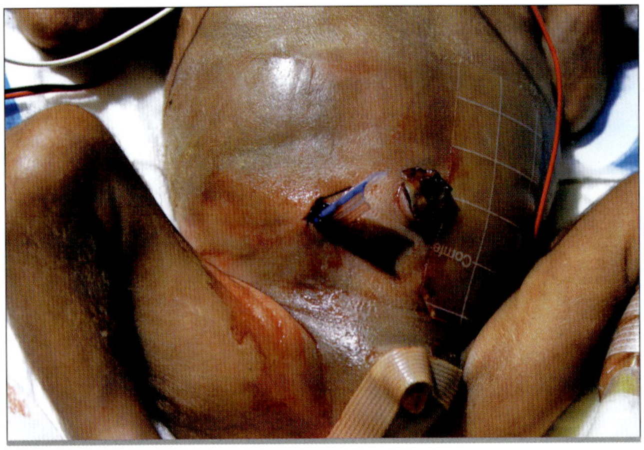

▸▸ **Fig. 12-6.** Penrose drainage of abdominal cavity in the case of intestinal perforation in an extremely-low-birth-weight infant.

13 Meconium Ileus

1) Etiology

Cystic fibrosis: extremely rare in Korean people

Intestinal obstruction by inspissated meconium

2) Classification

Simple or uncomplicated

Complicated: with intestinal perforation or necrosis

3) Clinical features (Fig. 13-1)

Same as those of intestinal obstruction or meconium peritonits

4) Diagnostic workup

- Plain abdomen (Fig. 13-2)
  - Dilated proximal bowel loops
  - "Soap bubble" in the right abdomen: air bubbles within meconium
- Contrast enema (Fig. 13-3)
  - With Gastrografin (hypertonic, water-soluble) or barium
- Sweat test
- Genetic test for cystic fibrosis

5) Differential diagnosis

Ileal atresia

Hirschsprung's disease

6) Nonoperative treatment

Hydration and nasogastric decompression

Gastrografin enema: diagnostic and therapeutic

7) Operative treatment

Enterotomy and evacuation of the meconium (Fig. 13-4)

Resection and anastomosis

Various forms of enterostomy

Exclude Hirschsprung's disease by histologic examination

Meconium Ileus

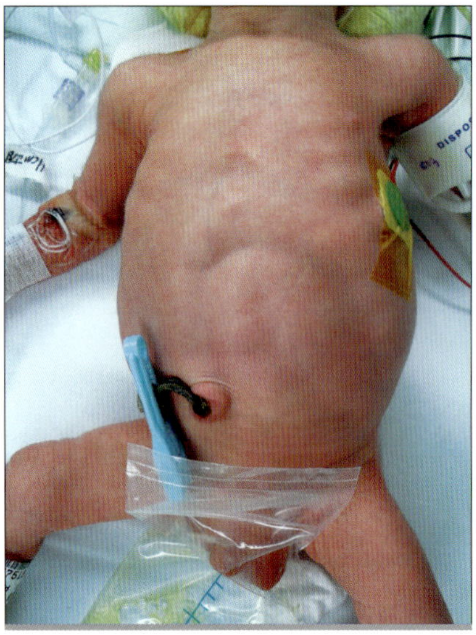

▸▸ **Fig. 13-1.** Abdominal distension with visible dilated bowel loops.

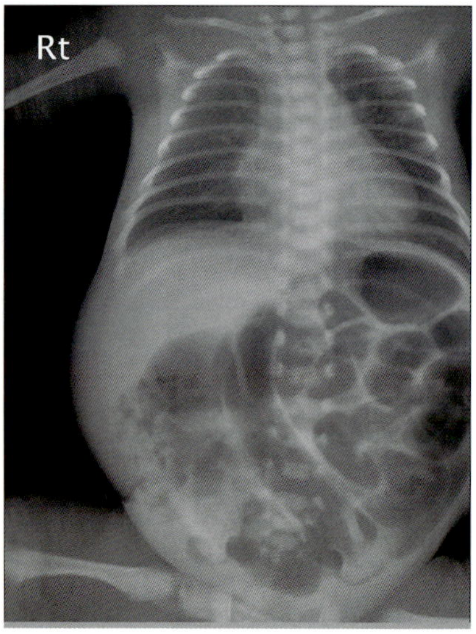

▸▸ **Fig. 13-2.** Plain film showing distended intestinal loops and "soap bubble" or "ground-glass" appearance in the right lower quadrant of the abdomen.

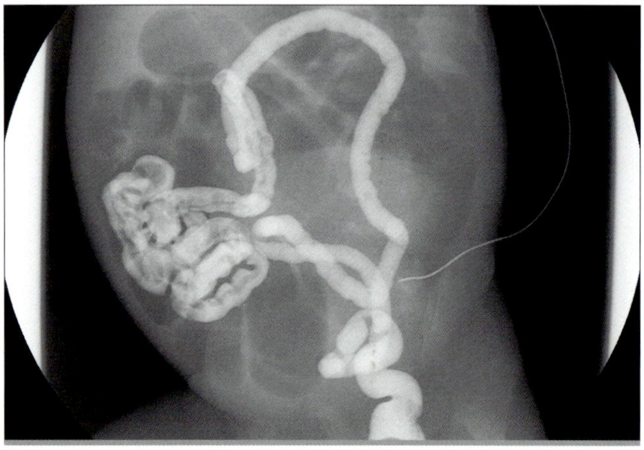

▸▸ **Fig. 13-3.** Gastrografin enema. The colon is of normal length but of small caliber (micro-colon) that is empty. The contrast refluxes into the proximal small bowel where pellets of inspissated meconium are outlined. The micro-colon can be seen in ileal atresia or total colonic aganglionosis. But, the contrast will not pass the atretic segment in ileal atresia. In total colonic aganglionosis, it will pass through the micro-colon into the dilated ileum without the pellets of inspissated meconium.

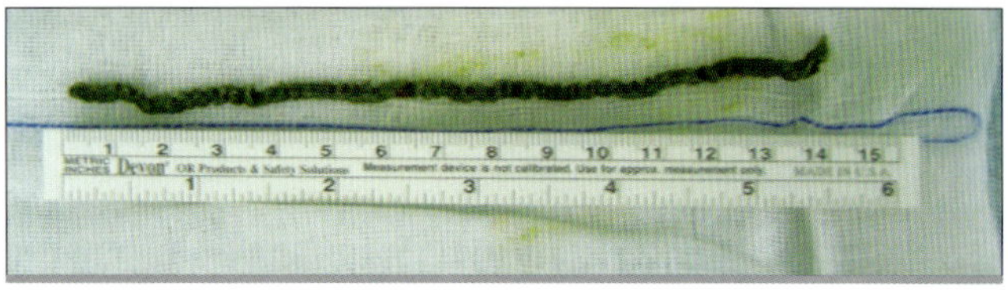

▸▸ **Fig. 13-4.** Pellets of inspissated meconium removed by operative enterotomy.

14 Necrotizing Enterocolitis

1) Etiology: uncertain

Ischemia and infection

Host immunity

2) Clinical features: Premature babies are more vulnerable.

Physiologic instabilities

Blood in the stool

Abdominal distension and bilious vomiting

Edema and erythema of the abdominal wall (Fig. 14-1)

Shock

3) Diagnostic workup

Plain abdominal film (Fig. 14-2)

- Pneumatosis intestinalis: pathognomonic
- Portal vein gas
- Fixed bowel loop
- Ascites
- Pneumoperitoneum: cross-table lateral film

4) Nonoperative treatment

Supportive care

Gastrointestinal decompression and nothing per os

Antibiotics for a minimum of 10 days

Careful serial examination

5) Operative treatment

Indications

- Absolute: pneumoperitoneum
- Other relative indications

Resection and anastomosis

Enterostomy - closed after a minimum of 4 to 8 weeks

Peritoneal drainage (Fig. 12-6)

6) Complication

Intestinal stricture

Necrotizing Enterocolitis

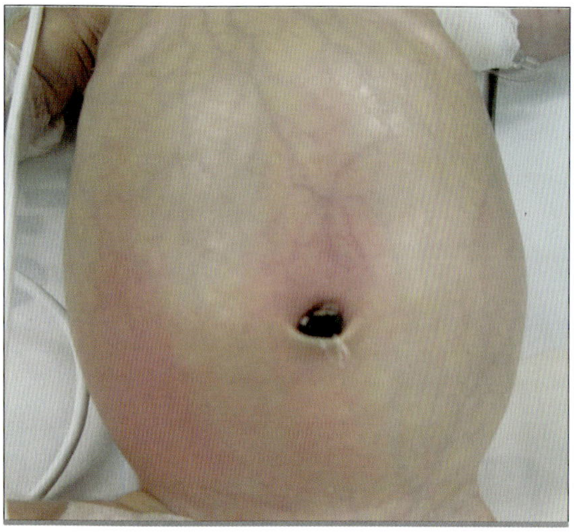

▸▸Fig. 14-1. Physical findings showing abdominal distension, erythema and prominent venous collaterals of the abdominal wall.

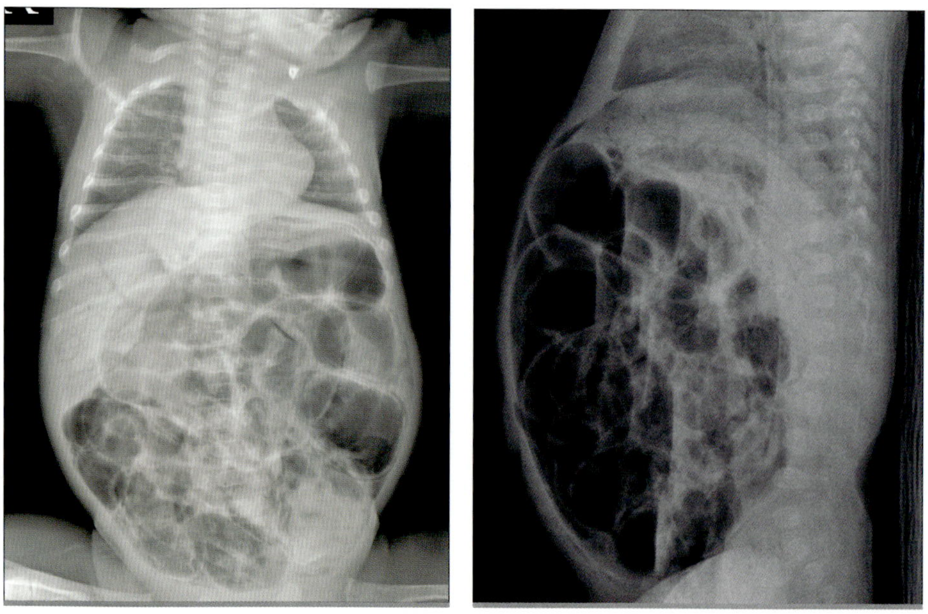

▸▸Fig. 14-2. Pneumatosis intestinalis, portal vein gas and pneumoperitoneum.

15 Intussusception

Invagination of one part of the intestine (intussusceptum) into another (intussuscipiens)

1) Etiology

Idiopathic: in more than 90%

Hypertrophy of Peyer's patches in the terminal ileum

Meckel's diverticulum, polyp, enterogenous cyst, etc.

2) Clinical features

Most commonly between 5 and 10 months of age

More common in male

A healthy infant suddenly begins screaming or awakens from sleep.

After a few minutes of attack, the baby appears normal.

The attacks usually occur every 10 to 15 minutes and are quite dramatic.

Bloody mucoid stool (Fig. 15-1), vomiting, lethargy

3) Diagnostic workup

Plain abdomen (Fig. 15-2): soft tissue density or features of intestinal obstruction

Ultrasonography (Fig. 15-3): target or kidney sign

Barium or air enema: diagnostic and therapeutic

4) Radiologic reduction: Air reduction is the preferred.

Pneumostatic reduction (Fig. 15-4 and 5) with air: maximum 120 mmHg

Easy to perform and more comfortable

Can be done quickly

Less radiation exposure

Repeated reduction possible

Less peritoneal contamination in case of bowel perforation

Hydrostatic reduction with barium: from 1m above the table

Ultrasound-guided saline reduction

5) Surgery

Indications

Peritonitis

Shock

Failed radiologic reduction

Intestinal perforation during radiologic reduction

Manual reduction (Fig. 15-6): milking backward of the lead point rather than pulling
Resection and primary anastomosis or enterostomy
Appendectomy is recommended.

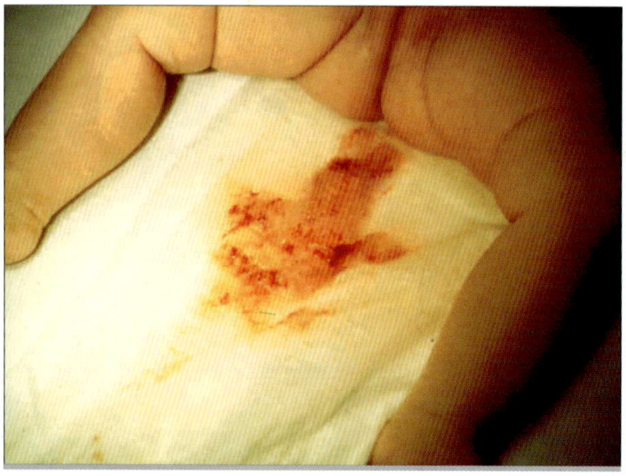

▸▸ **Fig. 15-1.** Bloody mucoid or currant jelly stool.

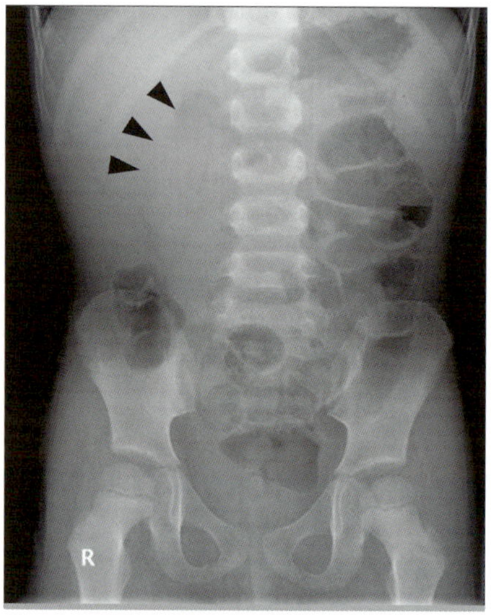

▸▸ **Fig. 15-2.** Plain abdomen showing soft tissue density (arrowhead) in the airless right upper quadrant of the abdomen.

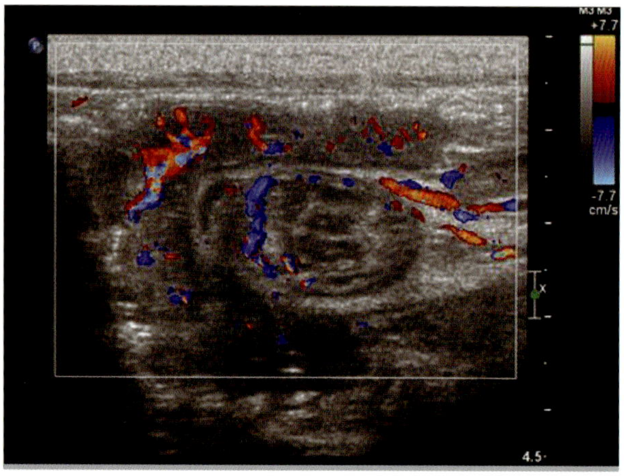

▸▸ **Fig. 15-3.** Target sign. Ultasonogram shows intussusception on cross section.

Intussusception

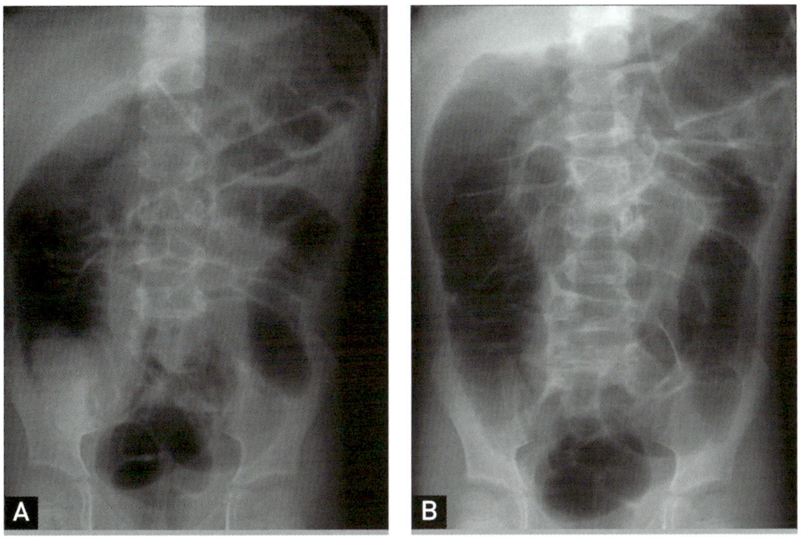

▸▸ **Fig. 15-4.** Air reduction. **A**, Intussusception is being reduced to the cecum. **B**, Intussusception is reduced successfully with reflux of air into the small intestine.

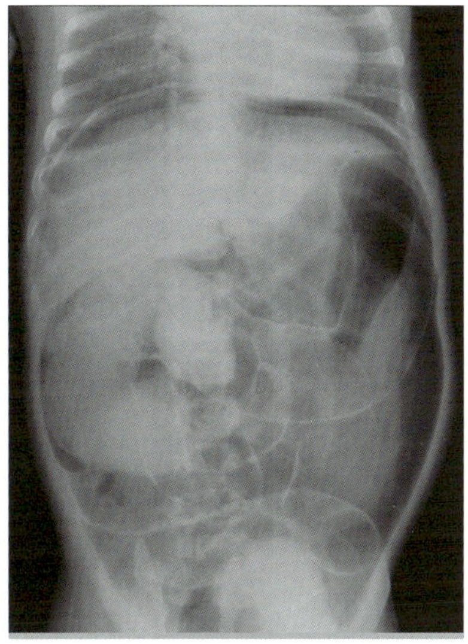

▸▸ **Fig. 15-5.** Pneumoperitoneum from perforation of the intestine during pneumostatic reduction.

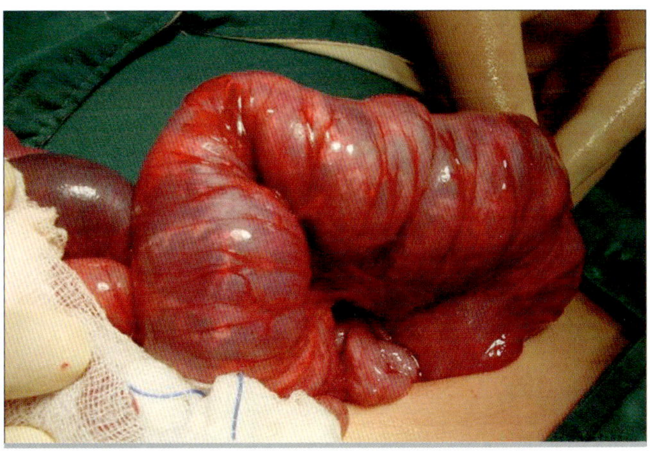

▸▸ **Fig. 15-6.** Manual reduction of ileo-sigmoid intussusception.

16 Alimentary Tract Duplication

1) Characteristics (William E. Ladd, 1937)

The presence of a well-developed coat of smooth muscle

An epithelial lining representing some portion of intestinal tract mucosa

Intimate anatomic association with some portion of the intestinal tract

2) Pathology

Cystic (Fig. 16-1) or tubular (Fig. 16-2)

Three fourths are cysts with no communication with the bowel lumen.

Mesenteric side (Fig. 16-1A), as opposed to Meckel's diverticulum

3) Clinical features

The majority of babies with duplications present in the first 2 years.

Partial intestinal obstruction

Abdominal pain, bleeding

Peptic ulceration (ectopic gastric mucosa)

Pressure effect to the adjacent structures (Fig. 16-3)

4) Diagnostic workup

Ultrasonography as a screening tool for abdominal cyst

Gastrointestinal contrast study

Endoscopy

Computed tomography

Magnetic resonance imaging

5) Surgery

Excision

Resection of intestine and anastomosis

Internal drainage at the distal end for long tubular duplication

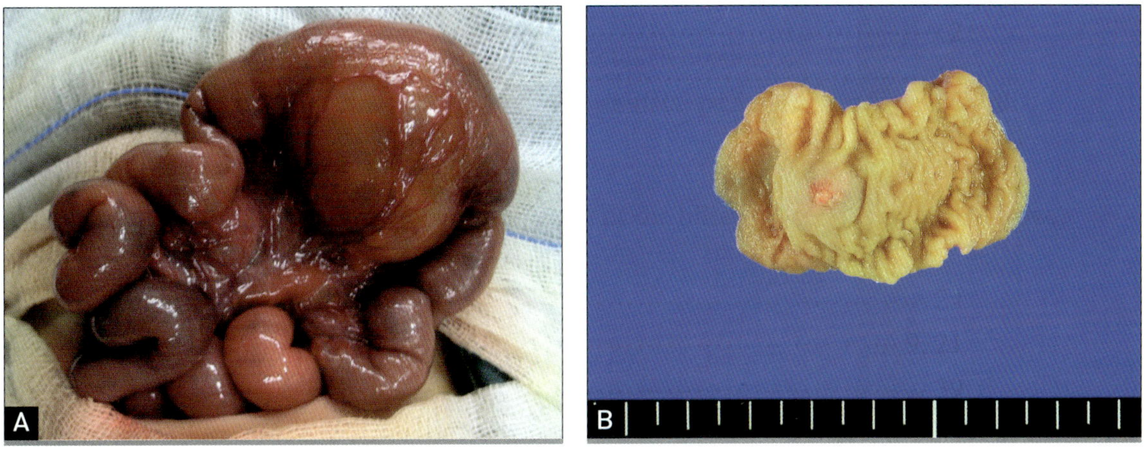

▸▸ **Fig. 16-1.** Cystic duplication of the small intestine. Note the cyst is on the mesenteric side **(A)** and communicates with the intestinal lumen **(B)**.

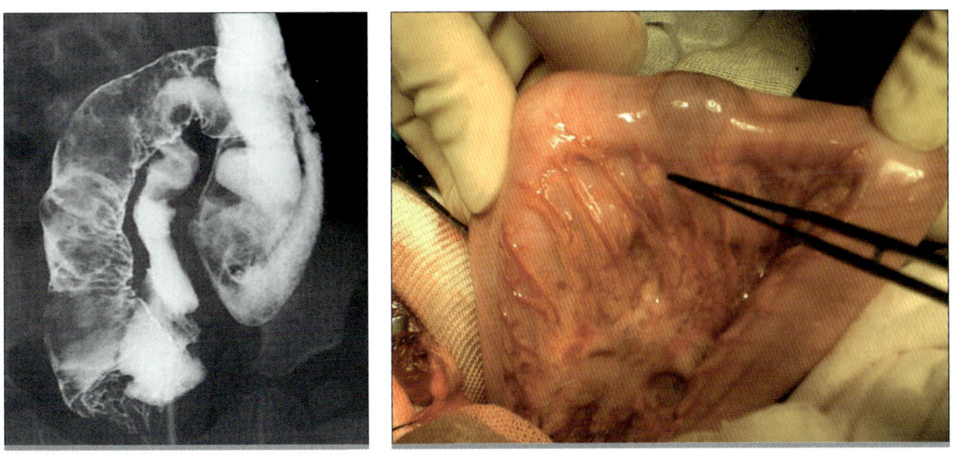

▸▸ **Fig. 16-2.** Colonic tubular duplication sharing a common wall.

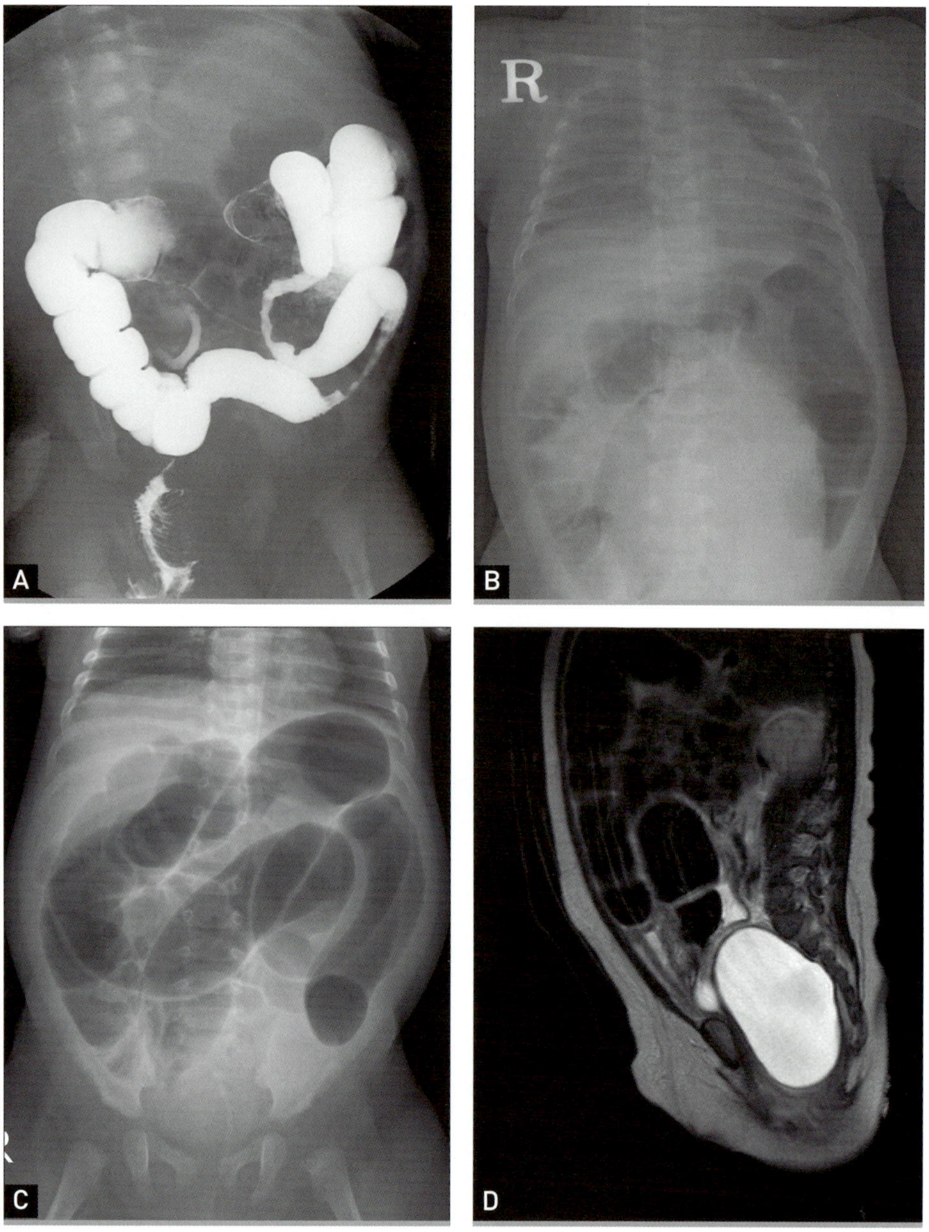

▸▸ **Fig. 16-3.** Rectal cystic duplication. **A**, Barium enema shows a submucosal mass in the rectum. **B**, Waiting elective operation, abdominal distension developed. Plain abdominal radiograph shows dilated intestinal loops and large soft tissue density in the middle to lower abdomen. **C**, The soft tissue density disappears after urinary catheterization but the dilated intestinal loops are still visible. **D**, MRI shows a large presacral retrorectal cyst compressing the rectum and urinary bladder.

17 Omphalomesenteric Duct Anomalies

1) Etiology

A failure of regression of vitelline duct between 5 and 7 weeks of gestation

2) Classification

Cyst

Sinus

Fistula (Fig. 17-1)

Meckel's diverticulum (Fig. 17-2 and 3): most common

3) Anatomy of Meckel's diverticulum

On antimesenteric border of the small bowel

True diverticulum containing all normal layers of the intestinal wall

Most are within 1m of the ileocecal valve.

Blood supply from primitive right vitelline artery arising directly from the mesentery (Fig. 17-2)

The right vitelline artery persists as the superior mesenteric artery and terminally supplies the diverticulum, but the left involutes.

Ectopic gastric mucosa in 60 to 85%

Ectopic pancreatic tissue in 5 to 16%

4) Clinical features: Only less than 5% of Meckel's diverticula are symptomatic.

Painless lower GI bleeding by

Peptic ulceration by ectopic gastric mucosa

Intestinal obstruction by

Prolapse through a patent vitelline duct

Volvulus around a fibrous band between diverticulum and umbilicus

Internal hernia beneath the aberrant right vitelline artery or a fibrous band

Intussusception

Inflammation (Fig. 17-3) and perforation

Similar to the features of acute appendicits

Related to the ectopic gastric mucosa or pancreatic tissue

Persistent umbilical granuloma, discharge from the umbilicus, abscess

5) Diagnostic workup

Fistulography (Fig. 17-4 and 5)

Technetium-99m pertechnetate isotope scintigraphy with pentagastrin (Fig. 17-6)

Isotope uptake by mucus-secreting gastric mucosal cells

Ectopic gastric mucosa (+) in 70% of symptomatic diverticula

6) Surgery

Diverticulectomy

Resection of the involved bowel

If ulceration (+) or ectopic tissue (+) at the diverticular base

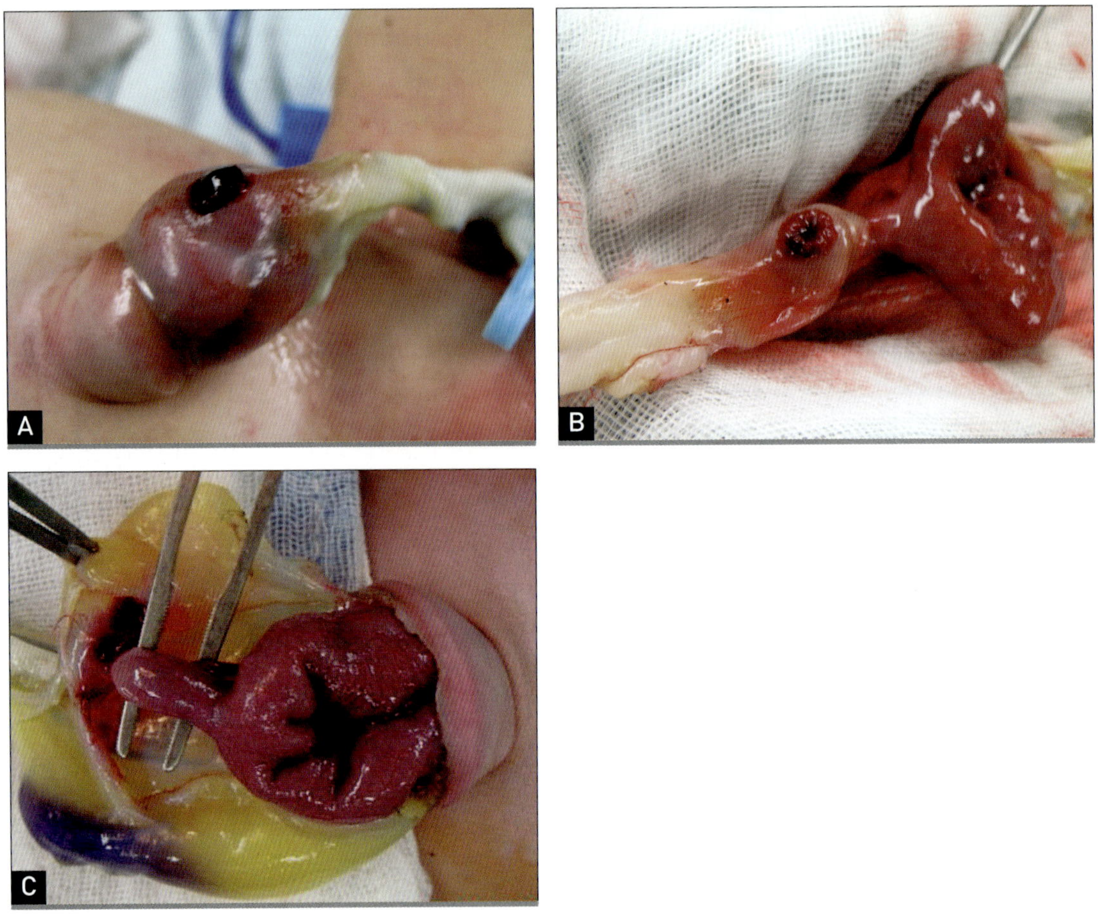

▸▸ **Fig. 17-1.** Patent vitelline duct with omphalocele. **A**, Meconium is observed on the sac of omphalocele. **B** and **C**, The fistula is between the antimesenteric side of the ileum and the top of omphalocele.

Omphalomesenteric Duct Anomalies

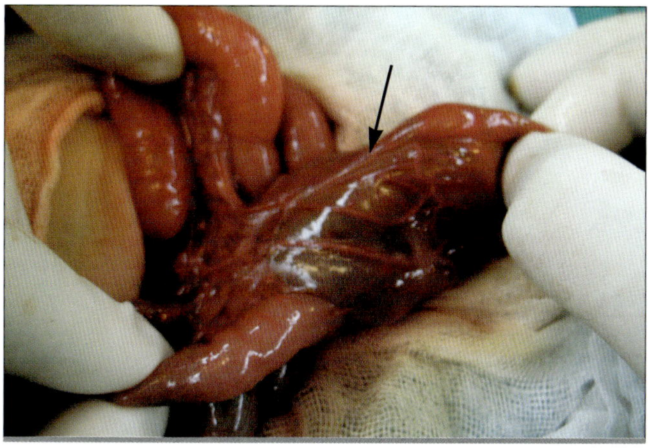

▸▸ Fig. 17-2. Meckel's diverticulum of antimesenteric side with an aberrant right vitelline artery (arrow).

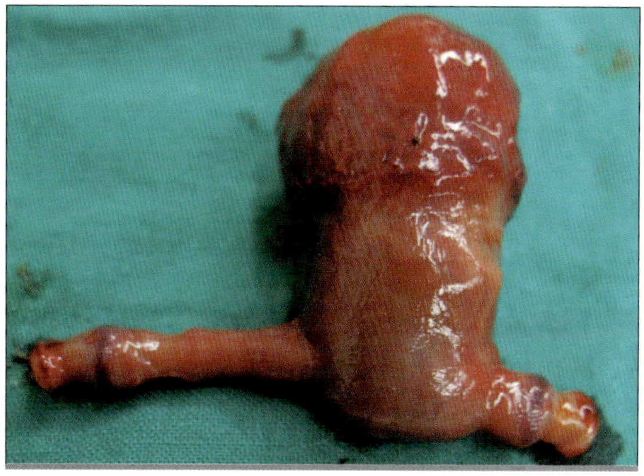

▸▸ Fig. 17-3. Meckel's diverticulum with inflammation.

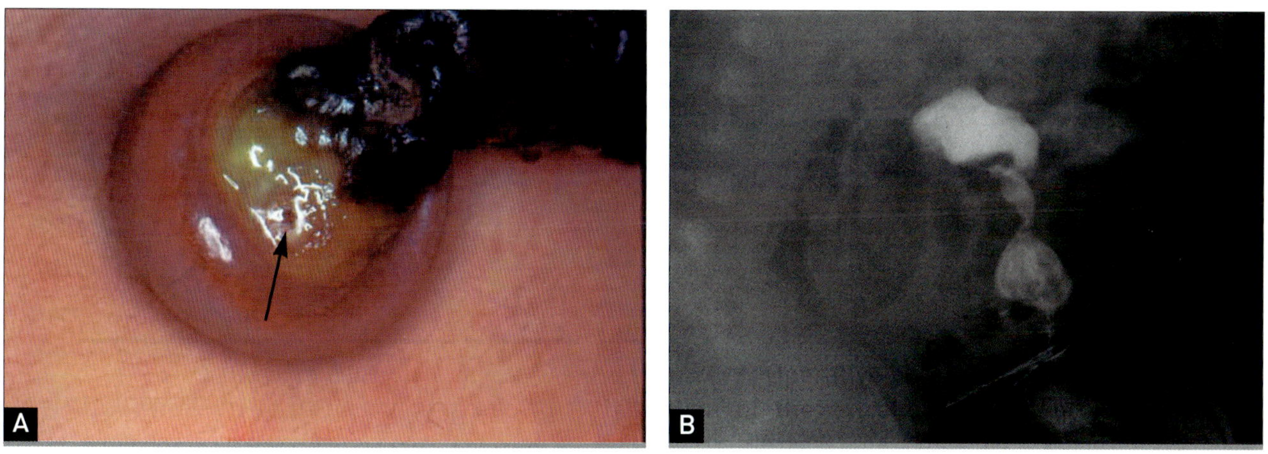

▸▸ Fig. 17-4. A draining opening **(A)** at umbilicus and fistulogram **(B)** showing the communication with the small bowel.

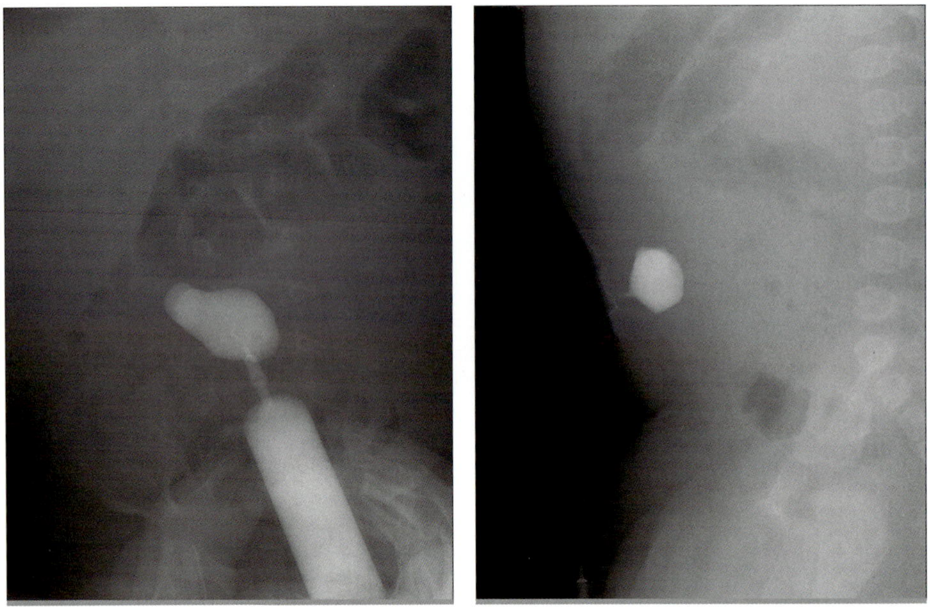

▸▸ **Fig. 17-5.** Contrast study of vitelline sinus. In addition to vitelline sinus, this baby had Meckel's diverticulum which was connected to the sinus by a fibrous band.

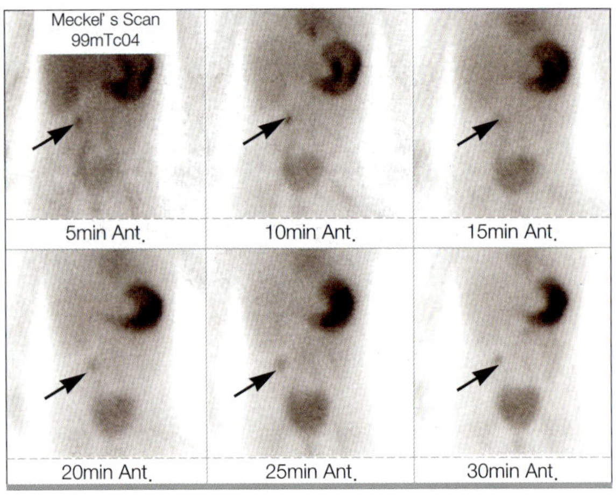

▸▸ **Fig. 17-6.** The diagnosis of Meckel's diverticum can be made by Technetium-99m scintigraphy if the diverticulum has ectopic gastric mucosa. The isotope activities are seen in the stomach, bladder. The abnormal uptake (arrow) is observed in the right side of abdomen suggesting Meckel's diverticulum.

18 Urachal Anomalies

1) Etiology

Persistence of the mucosa-lined lumen of the urachus extending from the bladder to the lower border of the umbilical ring

2) Classification

Cyst

Sinus

Bladder diverticulum

Patent urachus (Fig. 18-1 and 2)

3) Clinical fearures

Persistent draining

Infection and abscess

Mass

Cystitis

4) Diagnostic workup

Fistulography (Fig. 18-1)

Voiding cystourethrography (Fig. 18-2)

Ultrasonography

5) Surgery

Curvilinear infraumbilical incision

Complete excision to within a few millimeters of the bladder

Incision and drainage in abscess formation

Urachal Anomalies

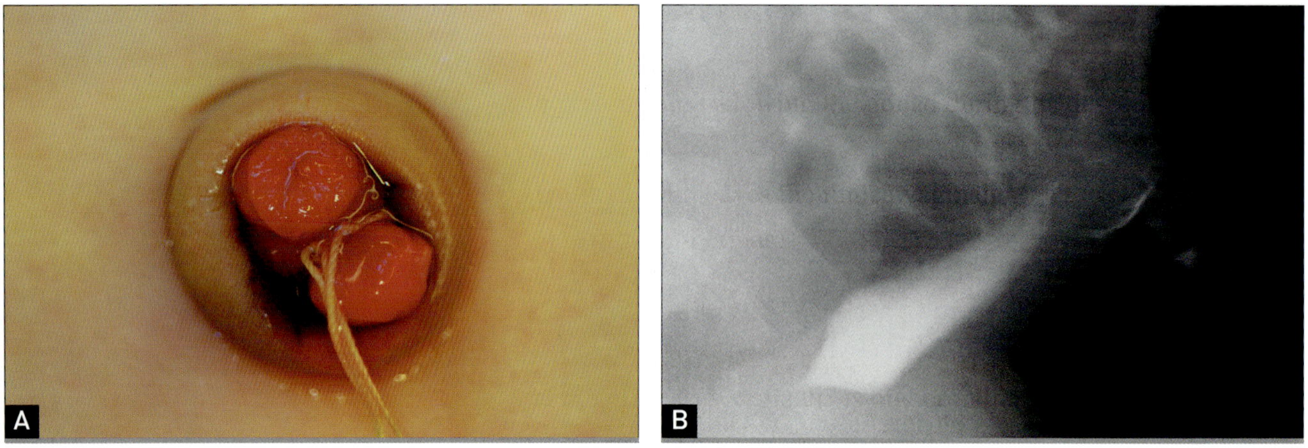

▸▸ **Fig. 18-1.** Patent urachus. **A**, After ligation-seperation of umbilical granuloma, a mucosa-lined opening was observed. **B**, Fistulogram through the opening reveals communication with the bladder.

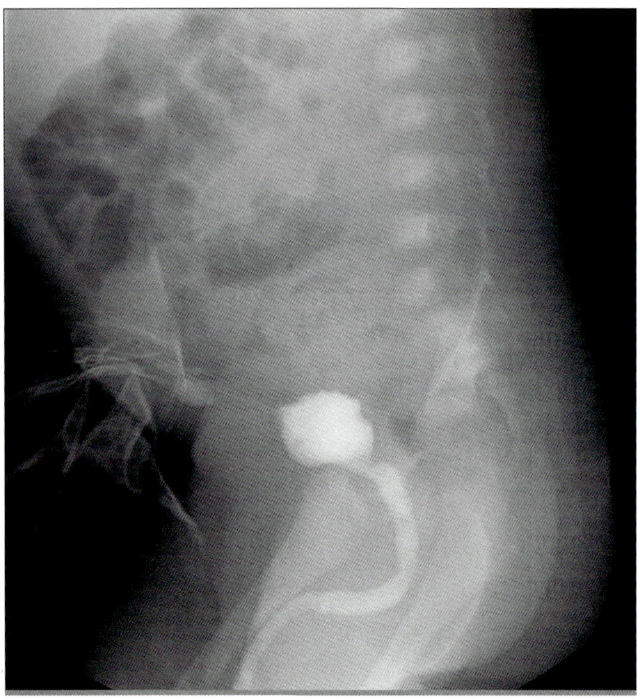

▸▸ **Fig. 18-2.** Patent urachus can be diagnosed by voiding cystourethrogram. The fistula draining to the umbilicus from the bladder is visualized.

19 Gastroschisis

1) Clinical features

Table 19-1. Characteristics of Gastroschisis and Omphalocele

	Gastroschisis (Fig .19-1)	Omphalocele (Fig .20-1)
Location	Right of umbilical cord	Umbilical ring
Defect size	Small	Large
Cord	Normal insertion	In sac
Sac	None	Present
Contents	Bowel	Bowel, liver
Bowel	Inflammed	Normal
Malrotation	Present	Present
Abdominal cavity	Small	Small
Associated anomalies	Uncommon (Bowel atresia in 10 to 15%)	Common, chromosomal

2) Prenatal treatment

The fetus and mother should be referred to the appropriate center.

Spontaneous vaginal delivery as close as possible to term is recommended.

3) Preoperative treatment

Alert hypothermia, hypovolemia, and sepsis

Prompt intubation with minimal ambu bagging, if needed

Nasogastric decompression

Meconium evacuation through anus

Prophylactic antibiotics

4) Surgery (Fig 19-2)

Primary reduction and repair, if possible

Silo formation and gradual reduction

Ventral hernia formation with prosthesis

Gastroschisis

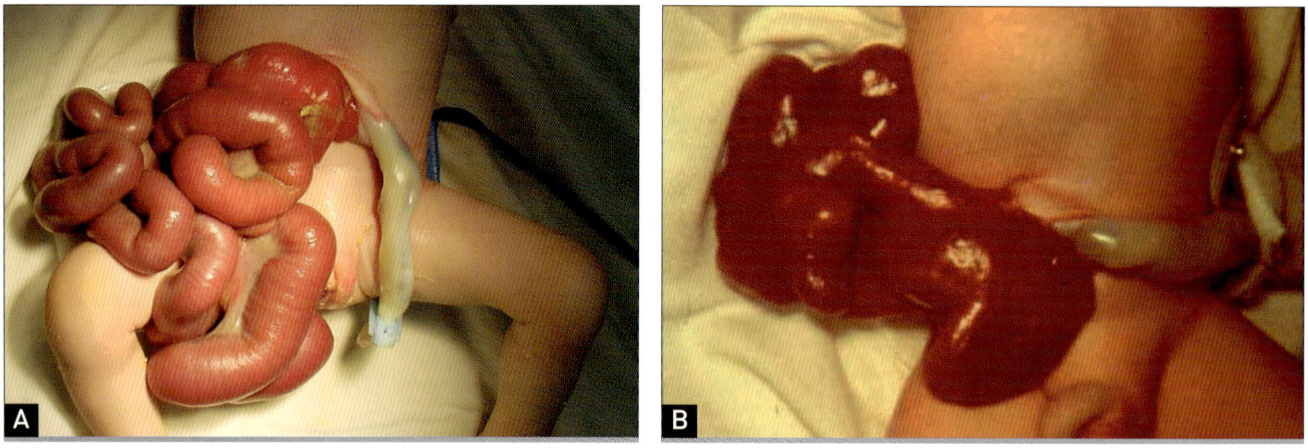

▸▸ **Fig. 19-1.** Gastroschisis. **A**, The small bowel is eviscerated through the small defect just to the right of a normal umbilical cord. There is no sac. **B**, The herniated bowel is edematous, glistening, and conglomerated because of the irritation of amniotic fluid.

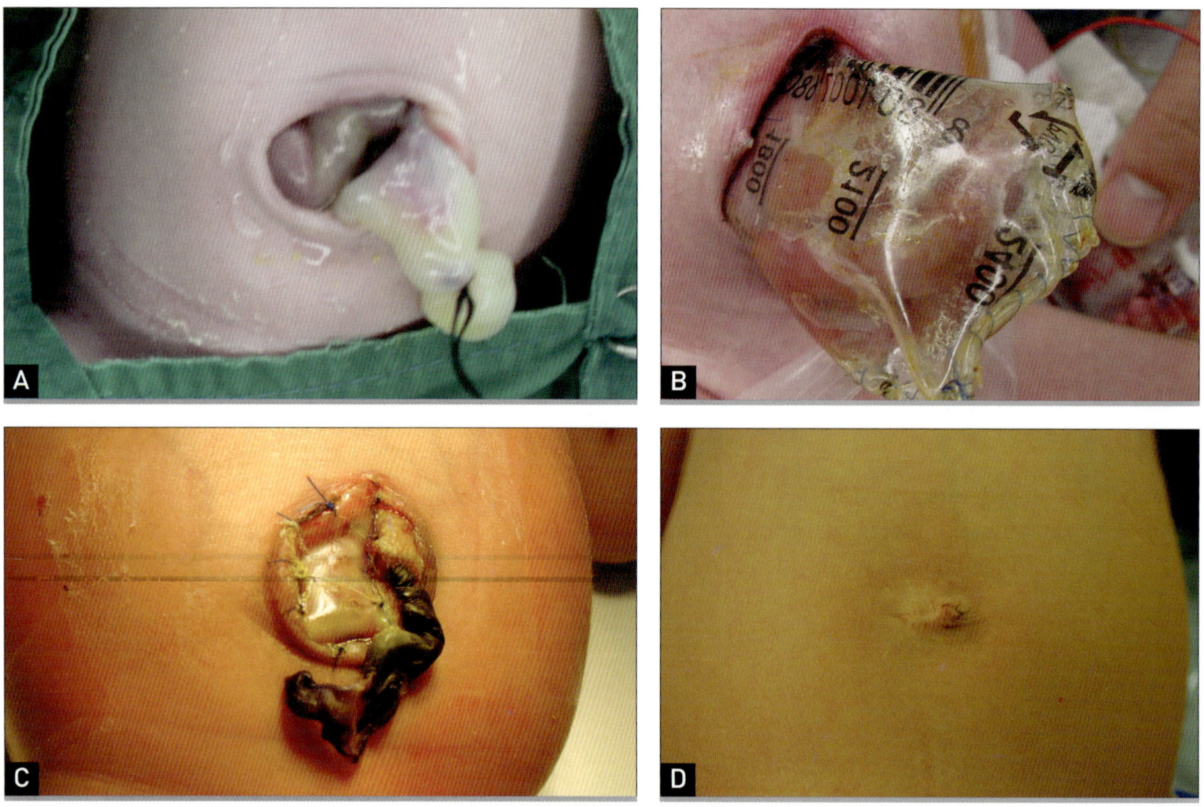

▸▸ **Fig. 19-2.** Repair of gastroschisis. **A**, The eviscerated bowel is reduced. **B** and **C**, When abdominal cavity is too small for the viscera, silo formation or patch closure is necessary. A saline bag can be a good temporary prosthesis. **D**, Good cosmetic result can be obtained by preserving the umbilicus.

20 Omphalocele

1) Clinical features (Fig. 20-1 and 2): See Table 19-1

Central omphalocele: a defect of the umbilical ring

Omphalocele in the epigastrium: pentalogy of Cantrell

- Omphalocele, epigastgric
- Anterior defect in the midline of diaphragm
- Defect in the lower part of pericardium
- Midline cleft of sternum
- Congenital heart disease

Omphalocele in the hypogastrium

- Bladder exstrophy
- Cloaca exstrophy (Fig. 20-3)

2) Prenatal treatment

The fetus and mother should be referred to the appropriate center.

Spontaneous vaginal delivery as close as possible to term is recommended unless the defect is too large.

3) Preoperative treatment

Prompt intubation with minimal ambu bagging, if needed

Nasogastric decompression

Protection of the sac

Meconium evacuation through anus

Prophylactic antibiotics

4) Surgery

Primary reduction and repair, if possible

Silo formation and gradual reduction (Fig. 20-4)

Ventral hernia formation with prosthesis

Escharotic agents application and delayed surgery

Omphalocele

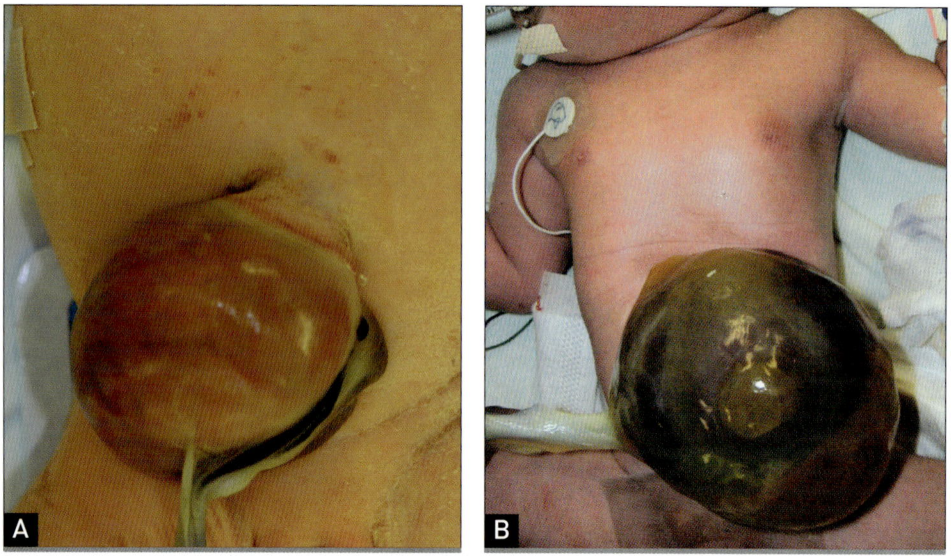

▸▸ **Fig. 20-1.** Omphalocele. **A**, The small intestine is herniated through the small umbilical defect with a sac. The cord inserts into the sac. **B**, Also, the liver is herniated through the large defect.

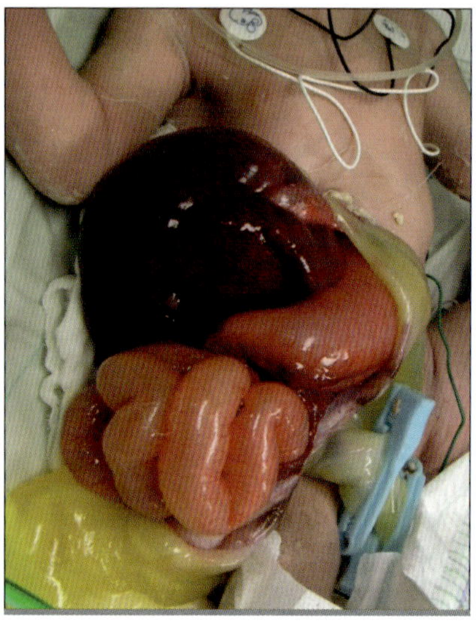

▸▸ **Fig. 20-2.** Ruptured omphalocele. The stomach, small intestine and liver are evicerated with the sac ruptured. The bowel is normal because the sac protects it from the irritation of amniotic fluid.

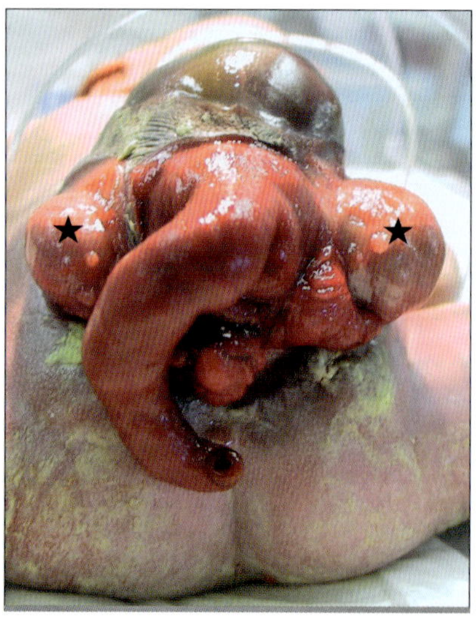

▸▸ **Fig. 20-3.** Omphalocele in the hypogastrium with exstrophy of the cloaca and imperforate anus. There are split bladder halves (asterisk) and a centrally located ileocecal plate with prolapse of the ileum.

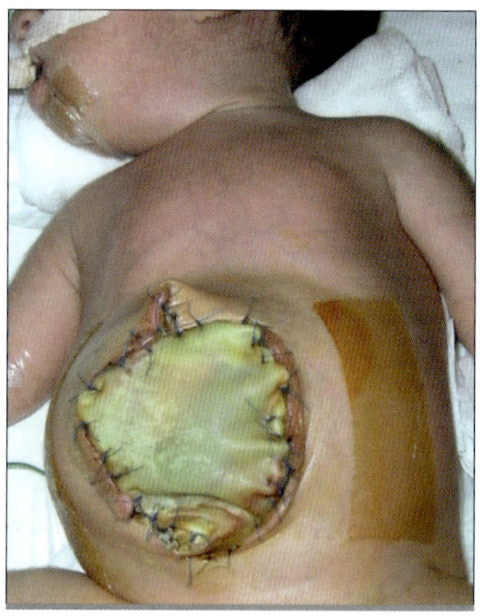

▸▸ **Fig. 20-4.** Prosthetic patch closure of epigastric omphalocele.

21 Hirschsprung's Disease

1) Etiology and pathophysiology

Arrest of the fetal development or cranio-caudal migration of the myenteric nervous system

→ Absence of ganglion cells in the intermuscular and submucosal plexus

→ Ineffective peristalsis of the aganglionic bowel

→ Functional obstruction

→ Dilatation and hypertrophy of the proximal normal ganglionic bowel

2) Clinical features

Aganglionosis is confined to the recto-sigmoid in 75% of the babies.

Abdominal distension

Failed meconium passage within 24 to 48 hours

Constipation and overflow diarrhea

Vomiting

Enterocolitis and sepsis

Rectal examination: empty rectum and gush-out of stool on withdrawal of the examiner's finger

3) Diagnostic workup

Plain abdominal films (Fig. 21-1) including cross-table lateral and pelvis lateral view

Barium enema (Fig. 21-2 and 3) without bowel preparation, and 24 to 48 hour delayed films

Anorectal manometry (Fig. 21-5)

Histologic examination

Full-thickness or submucoal suction rectal biopsy at 2 to 3 cm above the dentate line

4) Surgery

One or two stage operation

Leveling enterostomy at the transition zone (Fig. 21-4) in two stage operation

Resection of the aganglionic bowel: Swenson

Endorectal pull-through: Soave or transanal

Retrorectal pull-through: Duhamel

Hirschsprung's Disease

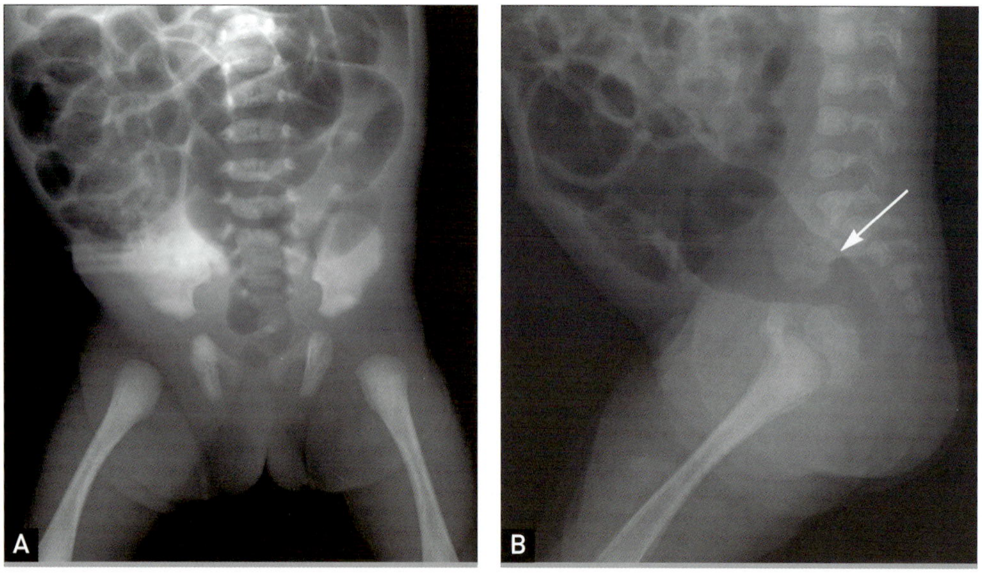

▸▸ **Fig. 21-1.** Plain abdominal films showing abdominal distension **(A)** and transition zone (arrow) in lateral view **(B)**.

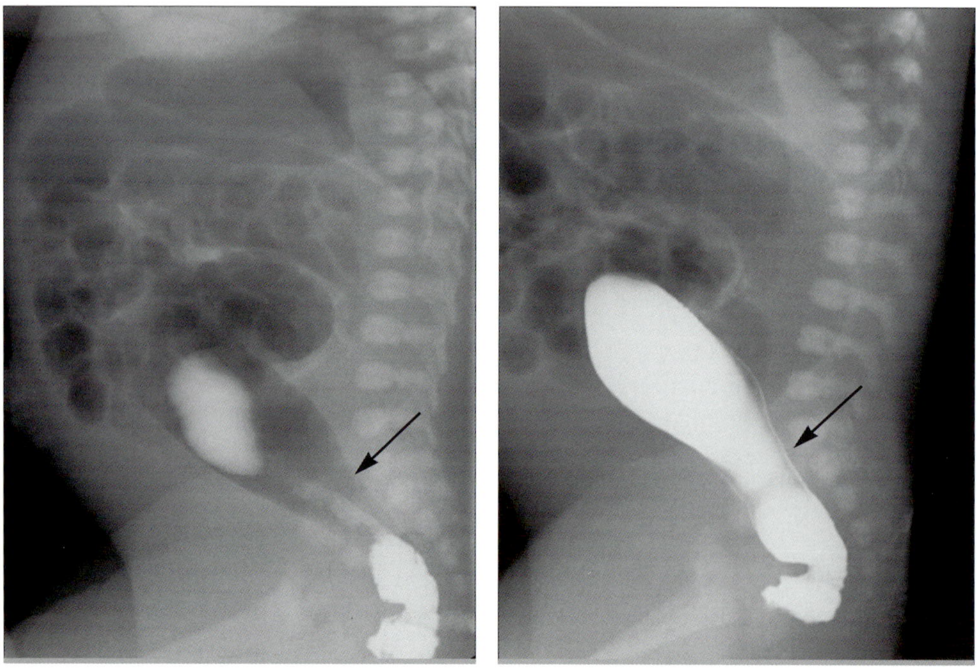

▸▸ **Fig. 21-2.** Barium enema showing transition zone (arrow). This study should be performed without prior bowel preparation and rectal examination. Lateral views of the rectum during filling in the absence of an inflated balloon catheter are important.

Hirschsprung's Disease

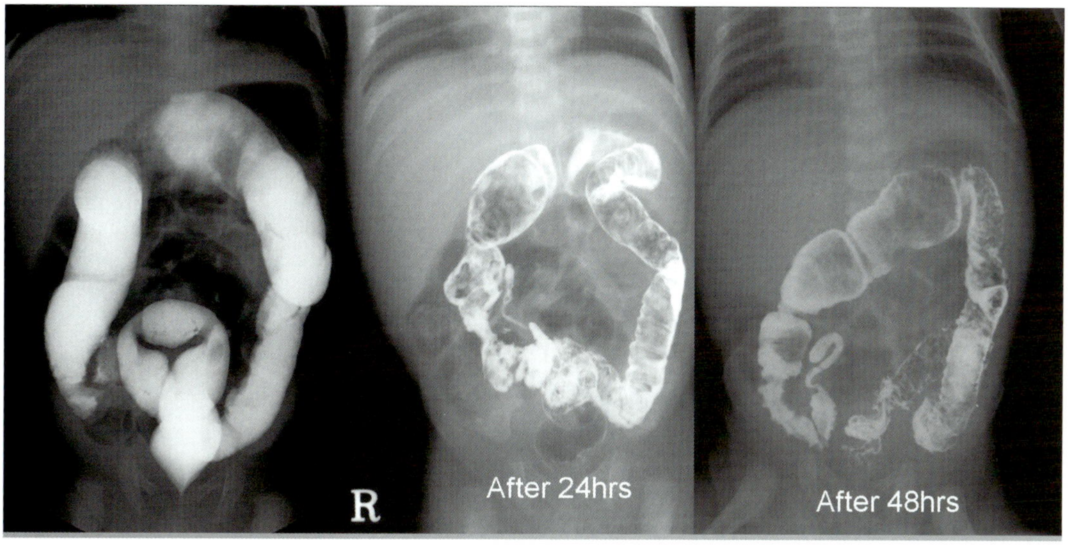

▸▸ **Fig. 21-3.** Total colonic aganglionosis. Bowel enema shows foreshortened colon without redundancy at flexures. There is no transition in the colon, but barium is retained even after 48 hours.

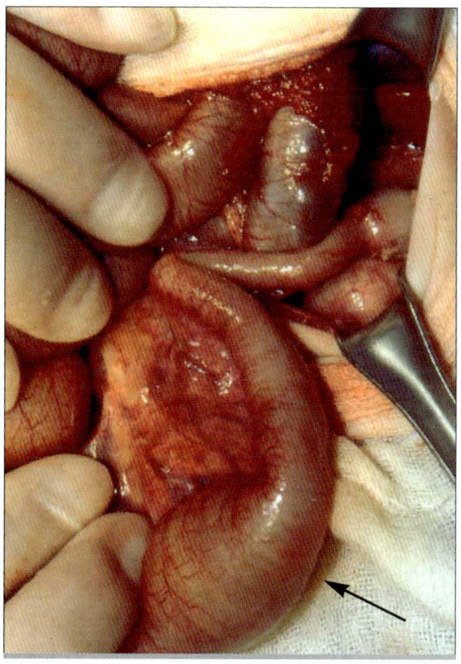

▸▸ **Fig. 21-4.** Transition zone (arrow) in the distal ileum.

Hirschsprung's Disease

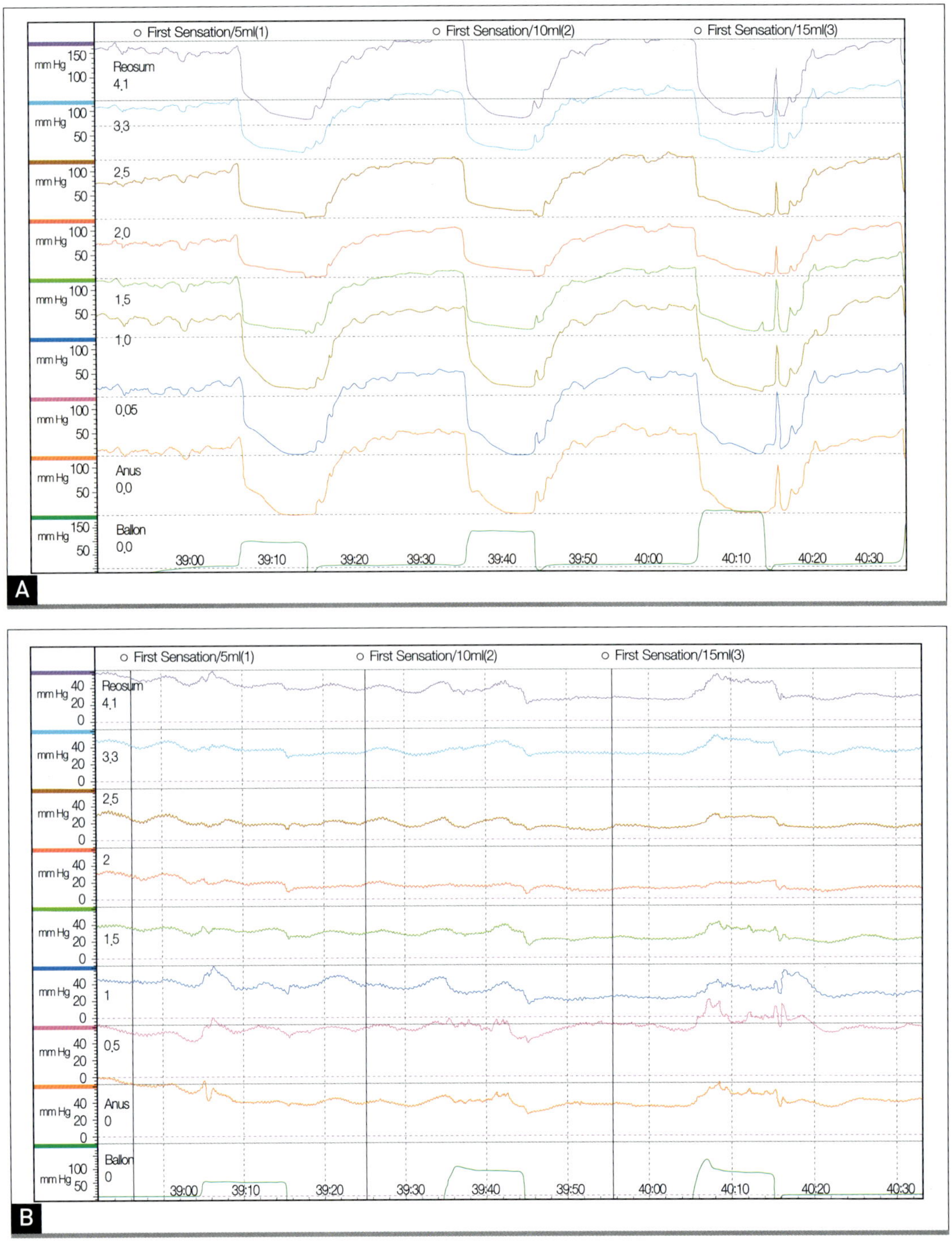

▸▸ **Fig. 21-5.** Anorectal manometry. **A**, Normal relaxation of the rectal sphincter in response to rectal distension is observed. **B**, In Hirschsprung's disease, the sphincter cannot relax in response to rectal distension.

22 Currarino's Triad

Sacral bone defect

Anorectal malformation, especially anorectal stenosis

Presacral mass: teratoma, lipoma, meningocele, or duplication cyst, etc.

1) Clinical features: familial in at least 50%

Constipation: most often

Perirectal abscess and fistula

Meningitis

2) Diagnostic workup

Plain lumbosacral spine film (Fig. 22-1 and 2)

Barium enema (Fig. 22-3)

Magnetic resonance imaging (Fig. 22-4).

3) Surgery: staged operation

(1) Diverting colostomy

(2) Neurosurgery, if needed for such as meningocele or tethered cord

(3) Excision of presacral mass and anorectoplasty through posterior sagittal approach

But, step (2) and (3) can be done simultaneously.

(4) Restoration of bowel continuity

Currarino's Triad

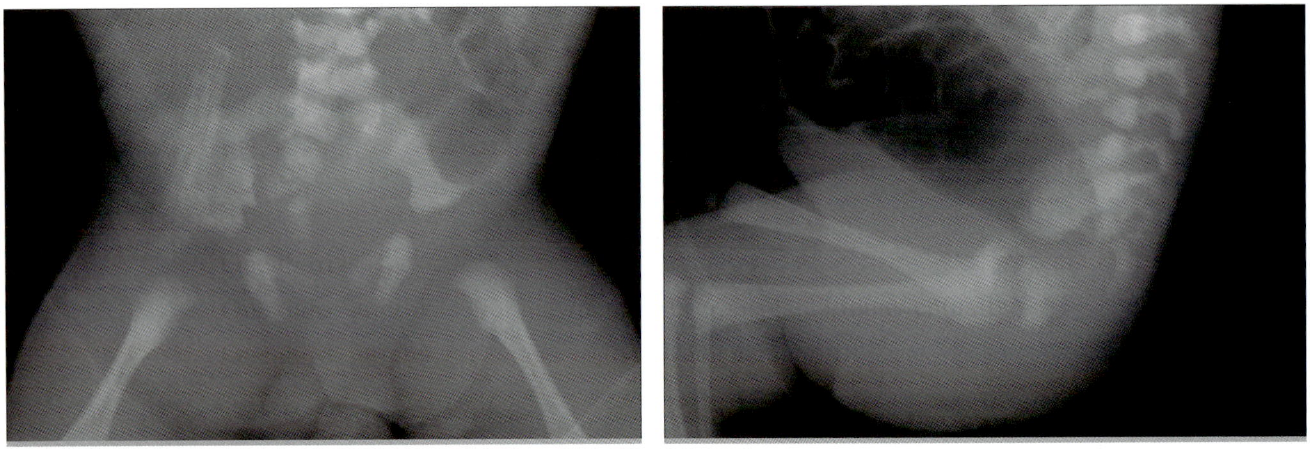

▸▸ **Fig. 22-1.** Currarino's triad. Bony defect of the left sacrum and rectal stenosis with proximal colonic dilatation are observed.

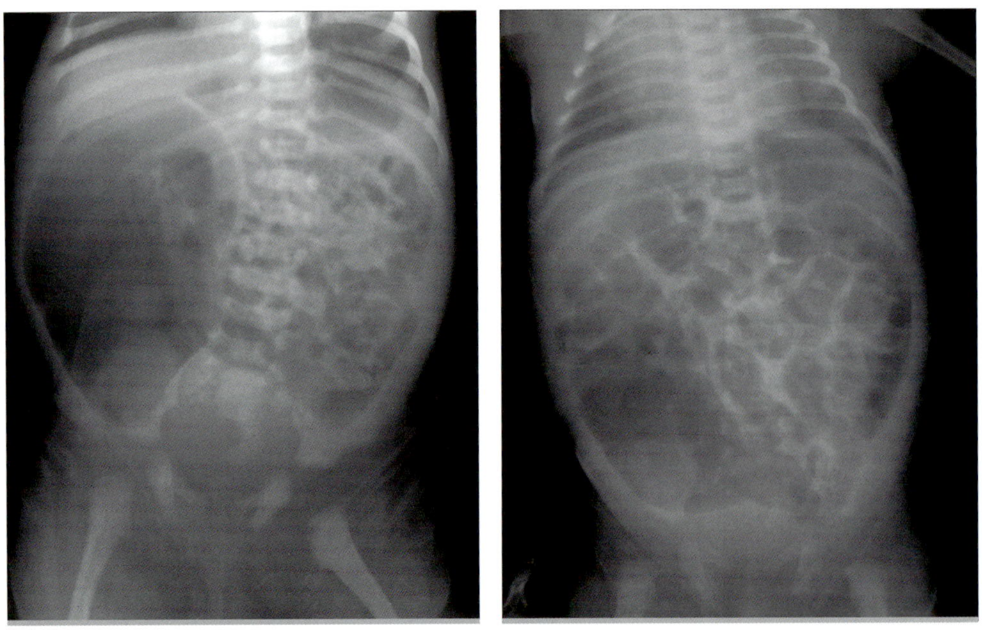

▸▸ **Fig. 22-2.** Plain films of Currarino's syndrome showing right-sided scimitar sacral bone defect with colonic dilatation.

Currarino's Triad

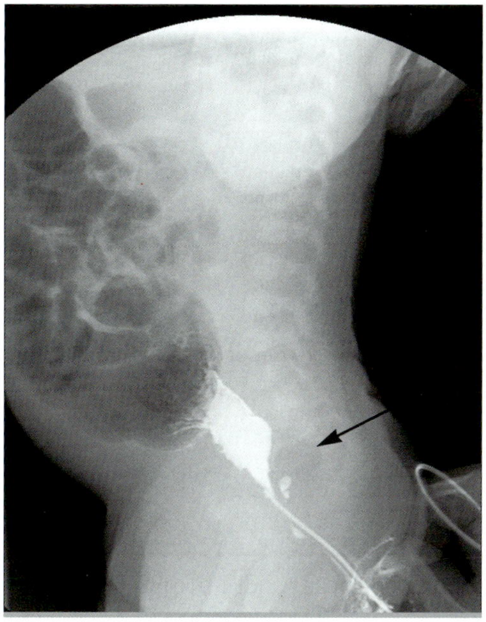

▸▸ **Fig. 22-3.** Contrast enema showing a radiolucent presacral space-occupying lesion (arrow) and rectal stricture. Sometimes the contrast from the bowel can be seen in the presacral mass, which increases the risk of infection.

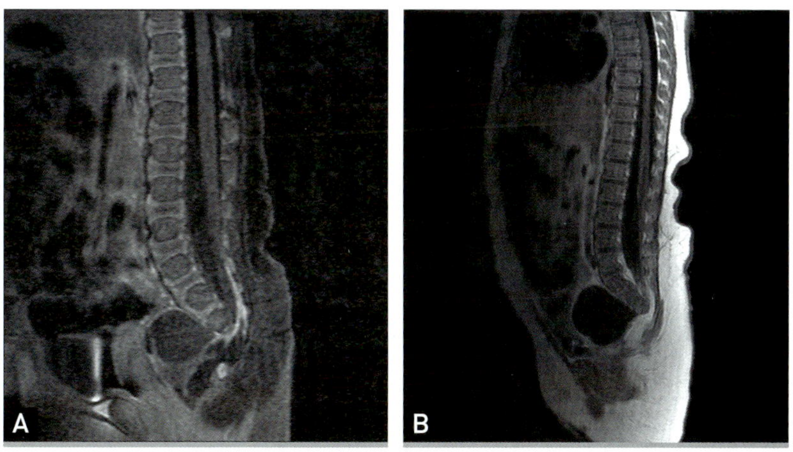

▸▸ **Fig. 22-4.** Magnetic resonance imaging showing presacral teratoma **(A)** and anterior meningocele **(B)** with tethered cords.

23 Anorectal Malformations (imperforate anus)

1) Embryology

The cloaca and cloacal membrane are present by the 4th week of gestation.

The cloaca receives the allantois, wolffian duct and the hindgut.

The urorectal septum grows downward, divides the cloaca from the above and finally joins the cloacal membrane,

The cloacal membrane breaks down at the 7th week, creating the urogenital and anal openings.

Failure of development of the posterior cloacal membrane results in various types of anorectal malformation.

Failure of development of the anterior and posterior cloacal membranes results in persistent cloaca anomaly with a common hindgut and urogenital opening.

2) Classification: Please refer to the articles for the schematic drawings.

Where is a fistula from the blind rectum?

Where is the blind rectum in relation to the puborectalis?

3) Clinical features

- Absence of the anus
- Membrane-covered or anterior-located stenotic anus (Fig. 23-1)
- Perineal fistula anterior to the anus (Fig. 23-2A and B)
- Meconium from the genitourinary system
    - Recto-urinary fistula in a boy (Fig. 23-3)
    - Recto-vaginal or -vestibular (Fig. 23-4) fistula or persistent cloaca (Fig. 23-5)
- Abdominal distension

4) Diagnostic workup: Whether is a colostomy required?

- Perineal inspection is most important.
    - Perineal signs (Fig. 23-2) of low type?
        - Meconium or epithelial pearl in the median raphe
        - Bucket handle deformity
    - Meconium in urine (Fig. 23-3)?
    - How many openings in the perineum in a girl?
        - 2 openings: recto-vaginal fistula
        - 1 opening: persistent cloaca (Fig. 23-5)
- Wait 24 hours to allow progression of gas or meconium down close to the perineum if the perineal signs of low type are negative.

5) Associated anomalies: VATER or VACTERL cluster

V: vertebral	- spine radiography (Fig. 5-7)
A: anal	
C: cardiac	- echocardiography
T: tracheal	- Chapter 5
E: esophageal	- Chapter 5
R: renal	- ultrasonography
L: limb	- inspection (Fig. 5-8)

6) Surgical treatment in a boy

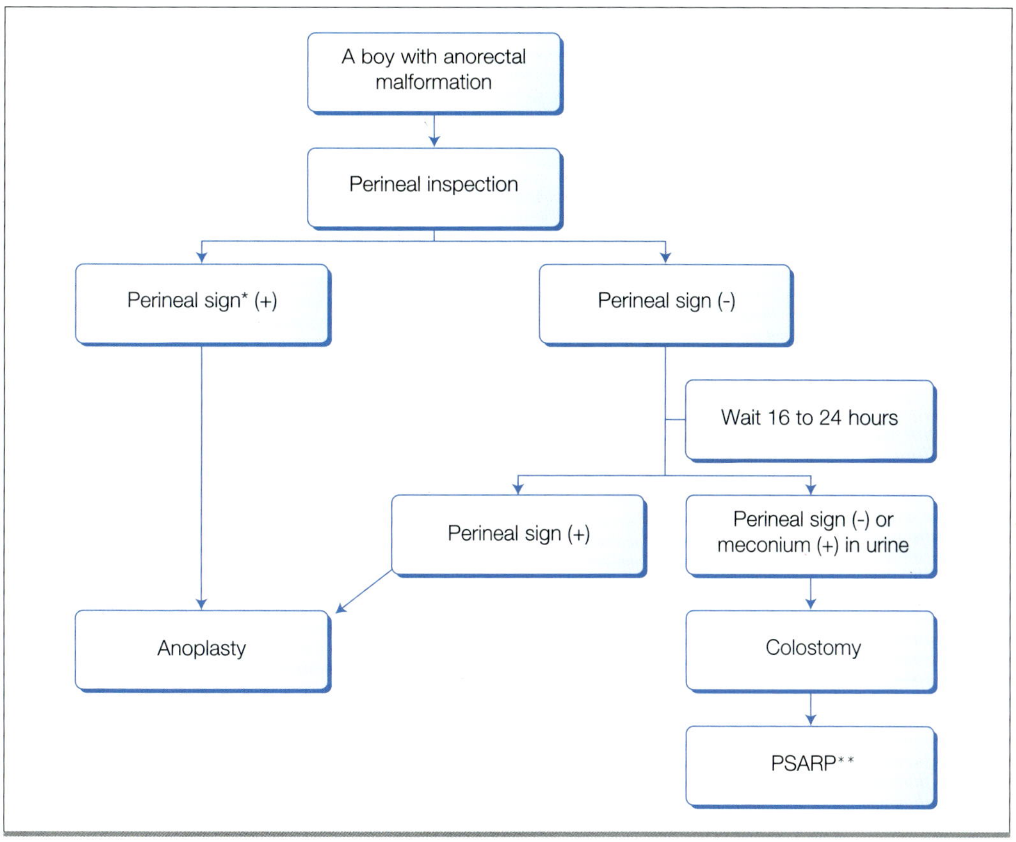

Algorithm for treatment of a newborn boy with anorectal malformation.
Perineal sign* includes meconium or epithelial pearl in the midline raphe and bucket handle deformitiy. PSARP** is posterior sagittal anorectoplasty.

Anorectal Malformations (imperforate anus)

(1) Low type

A) Anoplasty

Within the first 48 hours of life (before bacterial colonization of meconium)

Y-V advancement flap (Fig. 23-8) if necessary for the adequate size of the anus

B) Anal dilatation with a Hegar dilator (Fig. 23-6) from 2 weeks after surgery

Twice a day

Every week, the size is increased by one unit until the desired size is reached.

Once a day for 1 month

Twice a week for 1 month

Once a week for 1 month

Once a month for 3 months

Table 23-1. Size of Dilator According to Age

Age	Hegar dilator (No.)
1 to 4 months	12
4 to 8 months	13
8 to 12 months	14
1 to 3 years	15
3 to 12 years	16
More than 12 years	17

(2) High type

A) Colostomy

Descending or proximal sigmoid colostomy

to leave enough distal rectosigmoid for a future pull-through

The meconium in the distal colon should be removed.

B) Posterior sagittal anorectoplasty after distal loopography

Distal loopogram (colostogram) (Fig. 23-7)

The presence and site of rectourinary fistula

The distance from the rectum to anal dimpling

Urinary catheter for 5 to 7 days

C) Anal dilatation with a Hegar dilator from 2 weeks after surgery

D) Colostomy take-down when the correct size of the anus is reached

Anorectal Malformations (imperforate anus)

7) Surgical treatment in a girl

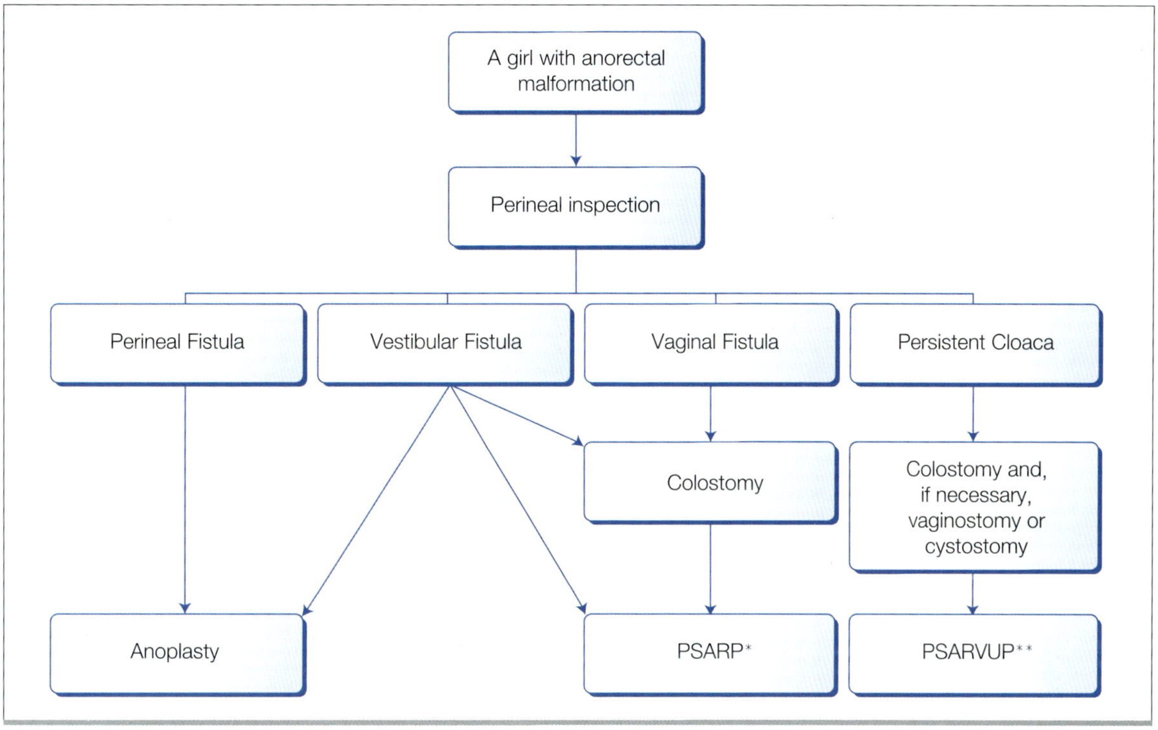

Algorithm for treatment of a newborn girl with anorectal malformation.
(PSARP*, posterior sagittal anorectoplasty; PSARVUP**, posterior sagittal anorectovaginourethroplasty)

8) Surgery

(1) Low type

A) Anoplasty (Fig. 23-8)

B) Anal dilatation with a Hegar dilator from 2 weeks after surgery

(2) High type

A) Colostomy

Vaginostomy or cystostomy may be needed in persistent cloaca (Fig. 23-9).

Hydrocolpos of mucous secretion can compress the trigone.

B) PSARP or posterior sagittal anorectovaginourethroplasty(PSARVUP)

Urinary catheter for 2 to 3 weeks in PSARVUP

C) Anal dilatation with a Hegar dilator from 2 weeks after surgery

D) Colostomy take-down when the correct size of the anus is reached

Anorectal Malformations (imperforate anus)

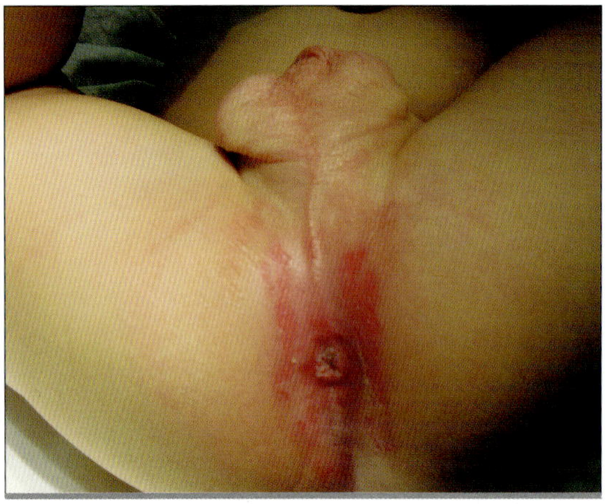

▸▸ **Fig. 23-1.** Anterior-located stenotic anus.

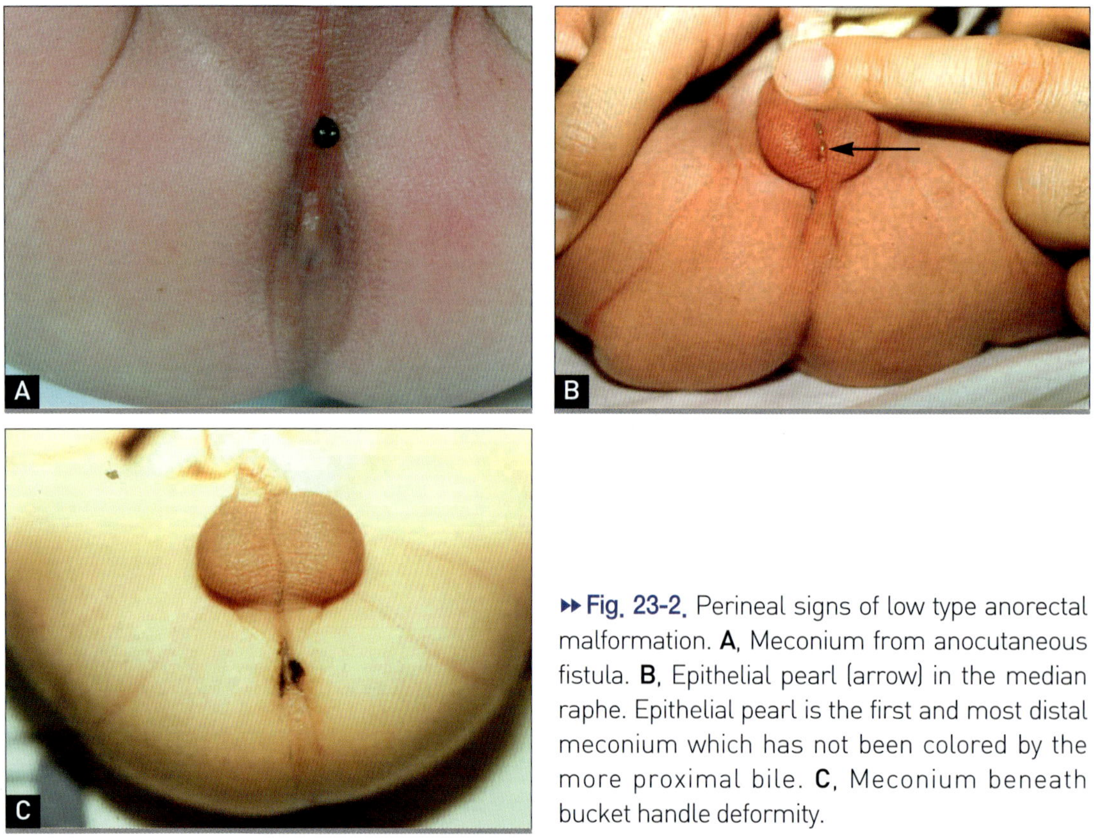

▸▸ **Fig. 23-2.** Perineal signs of low type anorectal malformation. **A**, Meconium from anocutaneous fistula. **B**, Epithelial pearl (arrow) in the median raphe. Epithelial pearl is the first and most distal meconium which has not been colored by the more proximal bile. **C**, Meconium beneath bucket handle deformity.

Anorectal Malformations (imperforate anus)

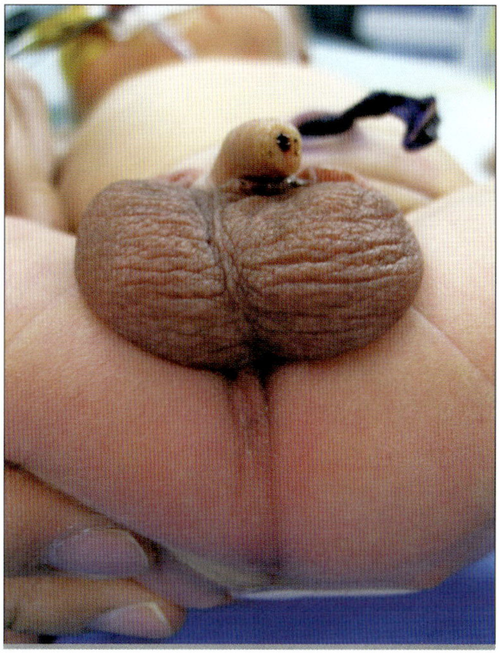

▸▸ Fig. 23-3. High type anorectal malformation. Meconium from the external meatus is observed, which suggests the presence of rectourinary fistula.

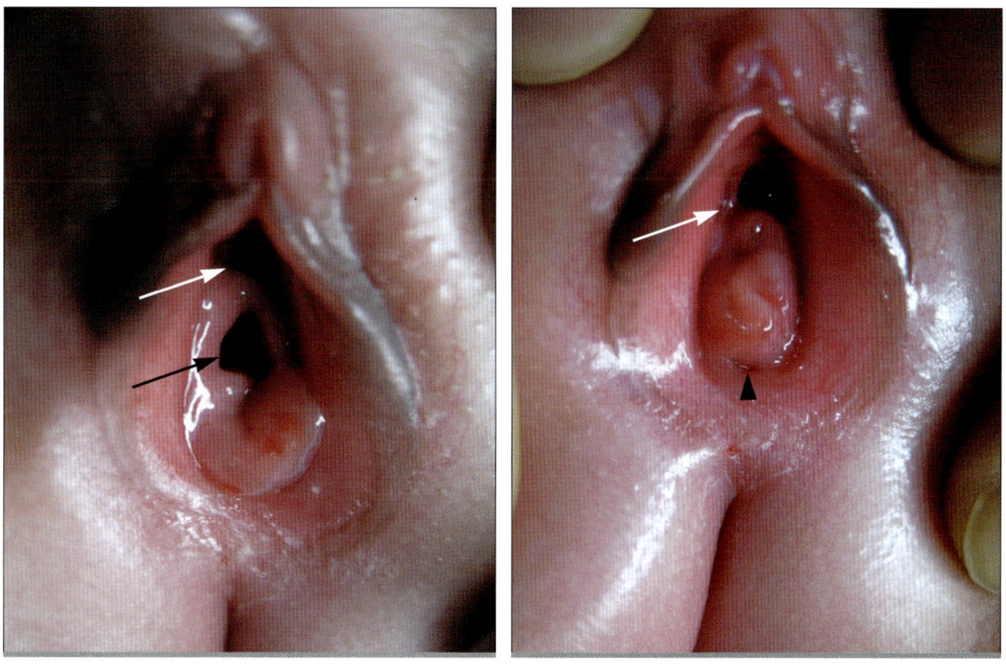

▸▸ Fig. 23-4. Rectovestibular fistula. Note the urethra (white arrow), vagina (black arrow) and vestibular fistula (arrowhead).

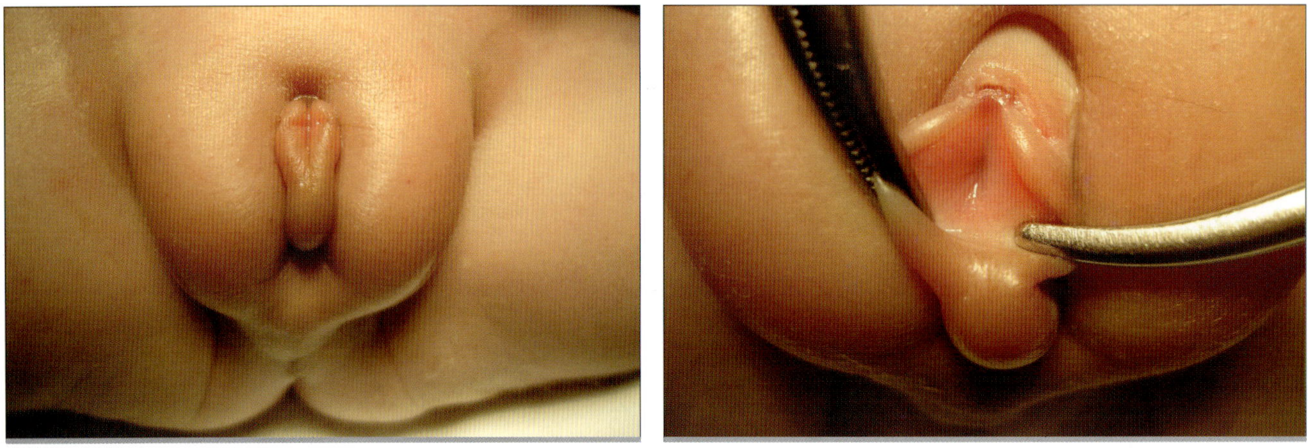

▸▸ **Fig. 23-5.** Persistent cloaca. The genitalia is small and separation of the labia discloses a single perineal orifice, a common opening for the urethra, vagina and rectum.

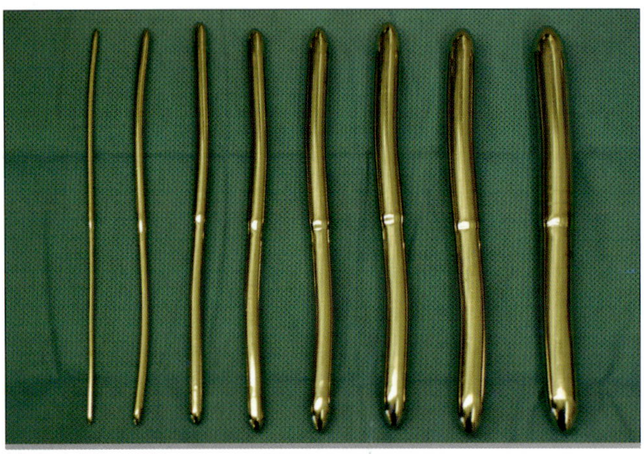

▸▸ **Fig. 23-6.** Hegar dilators

Anorectal Malformations (imperforate anus)

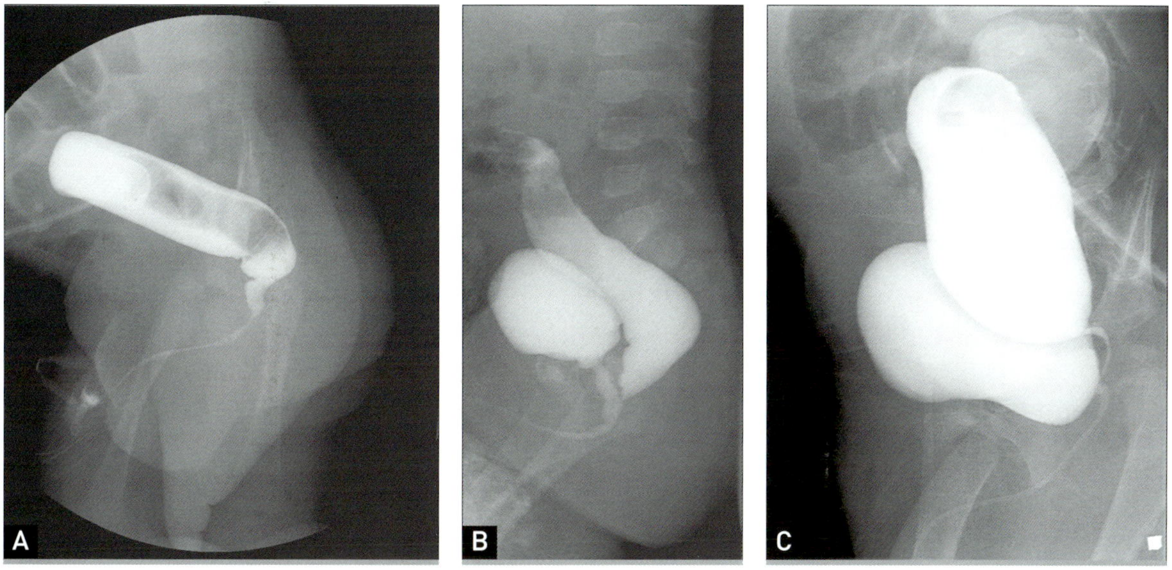

▸▸ **Fig. 23-7.** Diatal loopograms through colostomy showing recto-bulbous urethral fistula **(A)**, recto-prostatic urethral fistula **(B)** and recto-bladder neck fistula **(C)**.

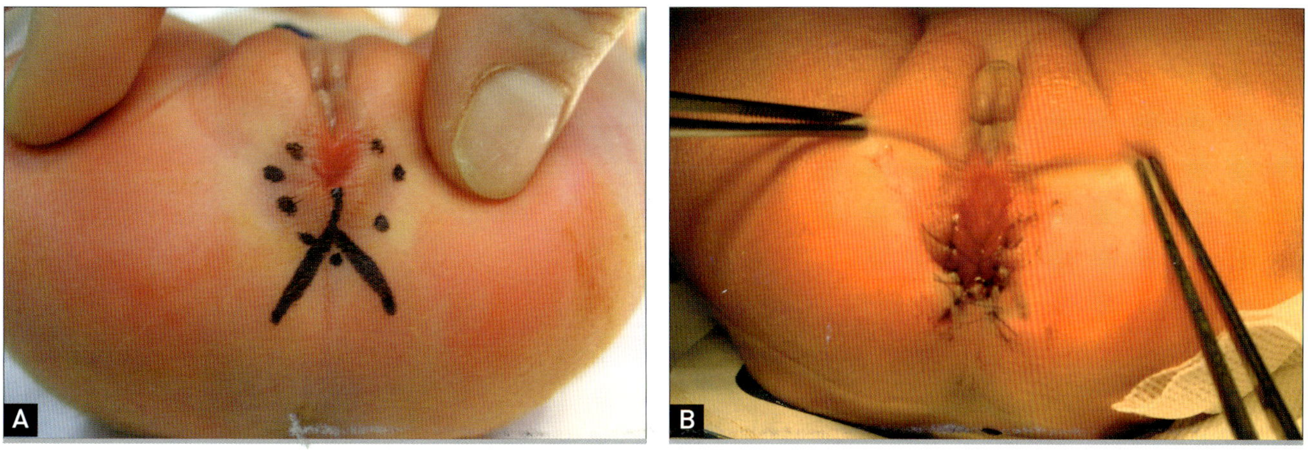

▸▸ **Fig. 23-8.** Y-V anoplasty. **A**, Inverted Y skin incision and a posterior skin flap are made. **B**, Midline incision in the rectal pouch is extended upward in the posterior rectal wall for incorporation of the inverted V-shaped advancement skin flap.

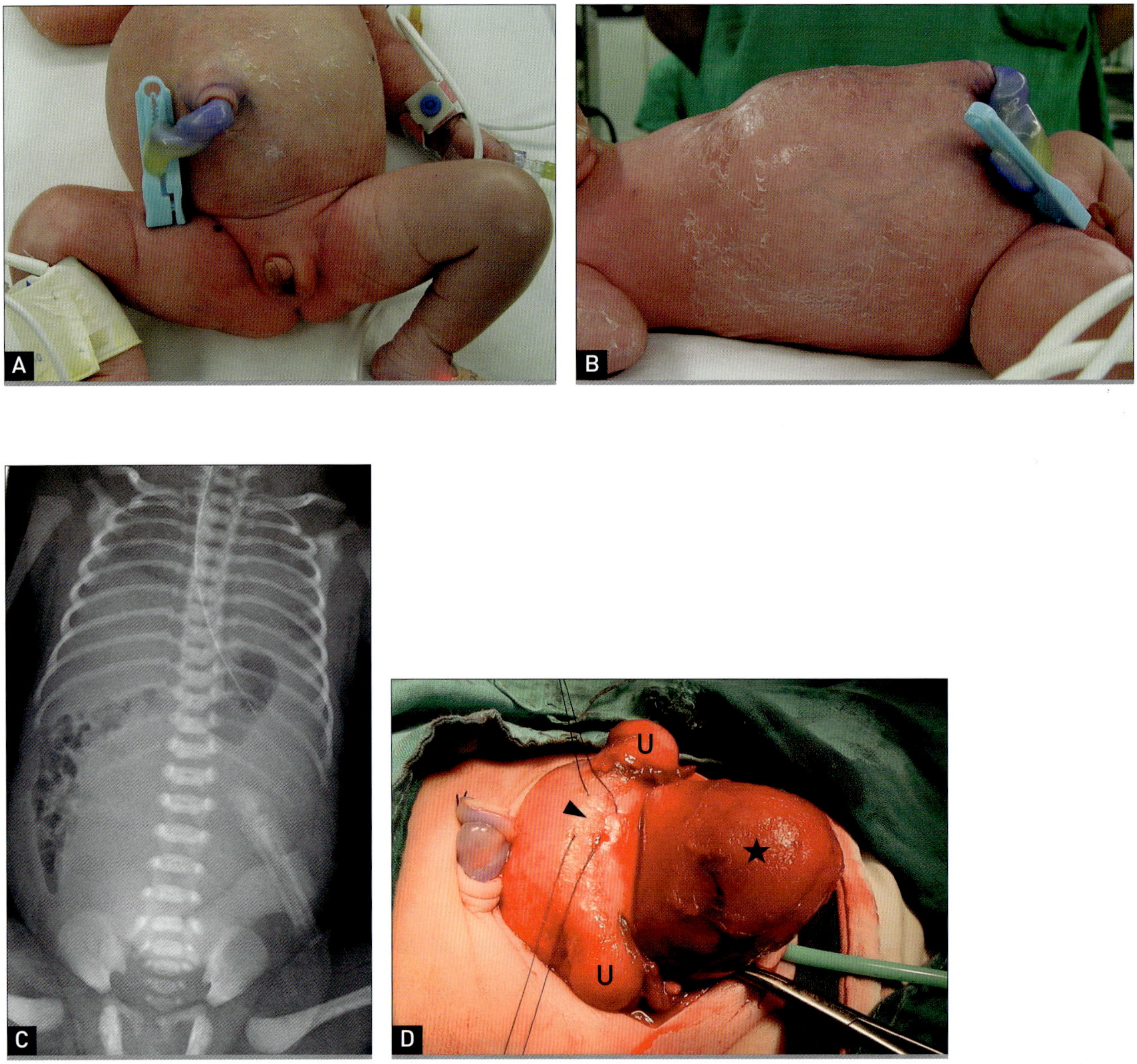

▸▸ **Fig. 23-9.** Persistent cloaca with hydrocolpos and megacystis (asterisk). **D**, Tube cystostomy is completed and tube vaginostomy (arrowhead) is ready. Double uterus (U) is observed.

24 Abdominal Lymphangioma

1) Clinical features

Abdominal pain, vomiting and mass

Sudden enlargement of a cyst with internal bleeding

2) Anatomy

Omental (Fig. 24-1), retroperitoneal (Fig. 24-2) or mesenteric (Fig. 24-3)

3) Diagnostic workup

Ultrasonography

Computed tomography

4) Surgery

Complete excision

Bowel resection in mesenteric lymphangioma

Partial excision and unroofing

Abdominal Lymphangioma

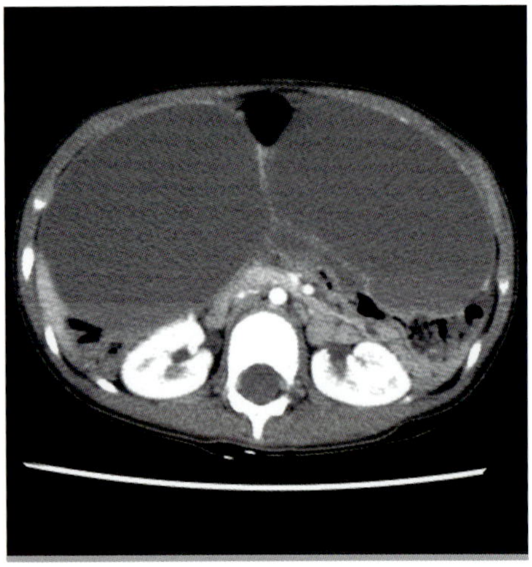

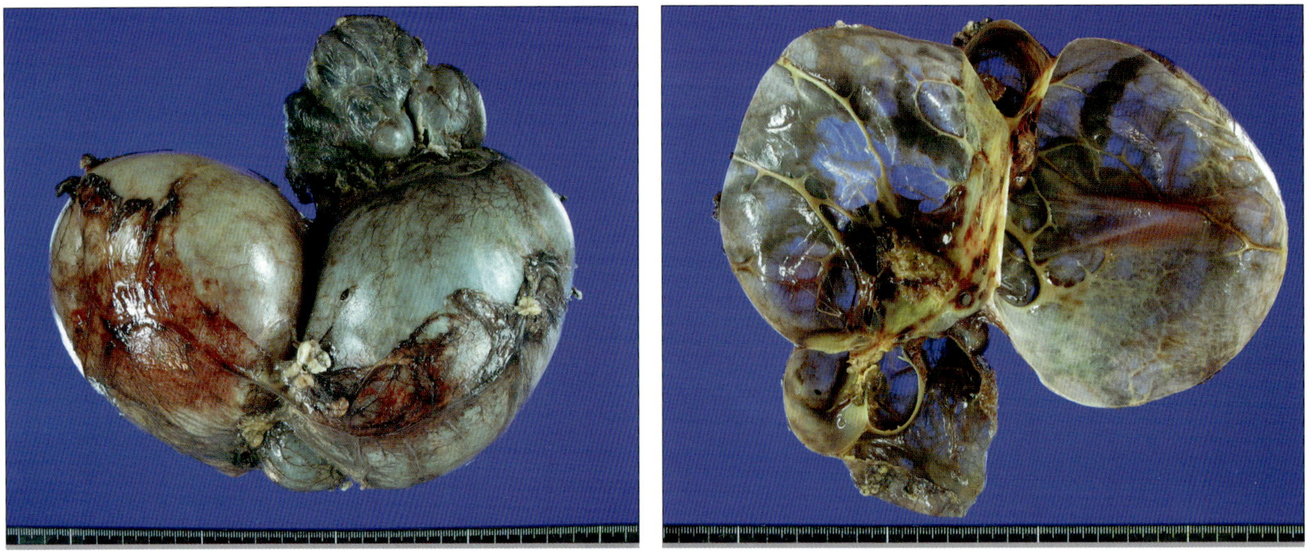

▸▸ **Fig. 24-1.** Omental lymphangioma made up of large cysts.

Abdominal Lymphangioma

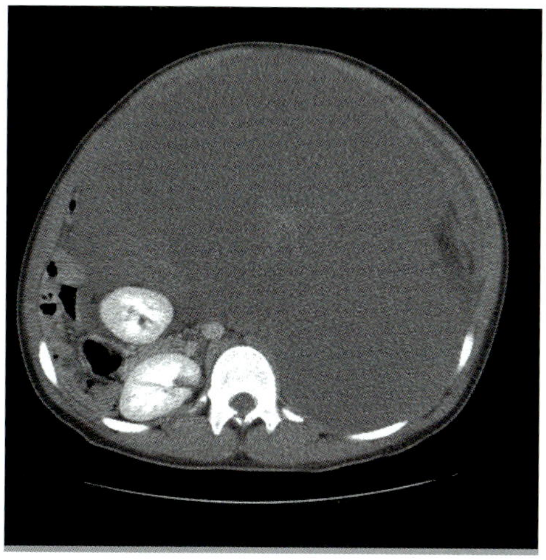

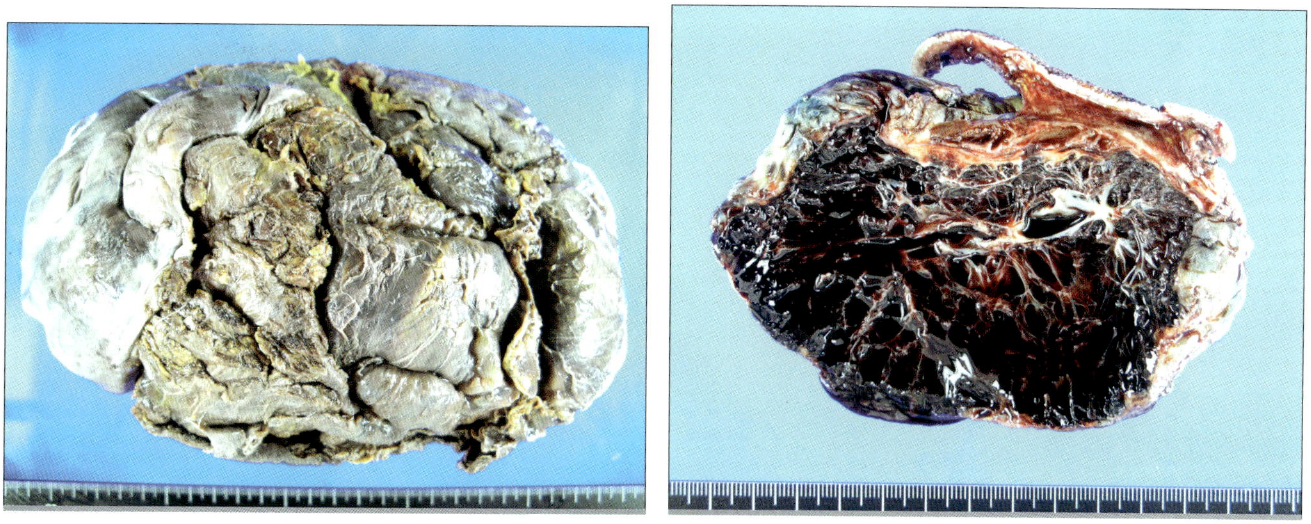

▸▸**Fig. 24-2.** Retroperitoneal lymphangioma. The left kidney is displaced to the right adjacent to the right kidney. The mass consists of multiple small cysts with internal bleeding.

Abdominal Lymphangioma

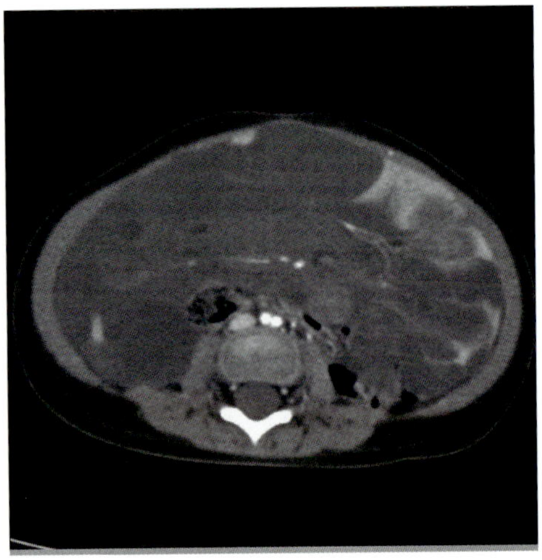

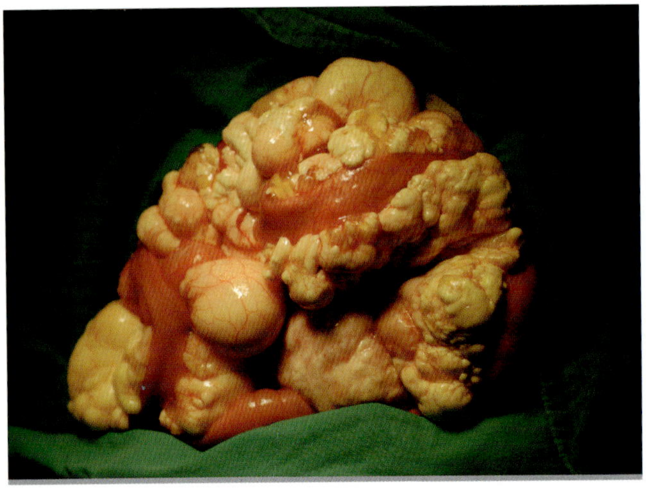

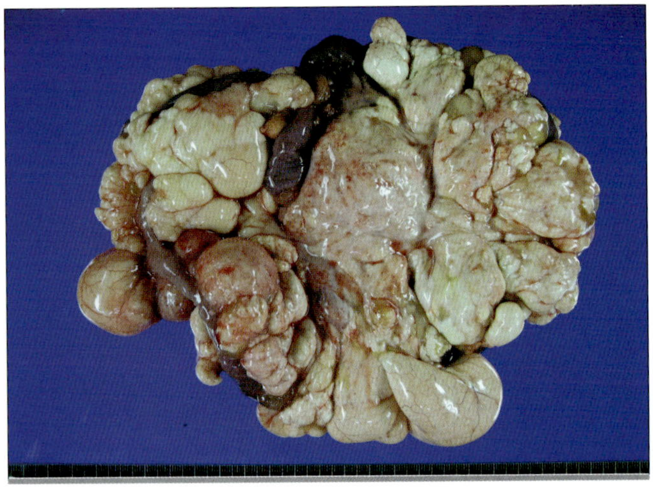

▸▸ **Fig. 24-3.** Mesenteric lymphangioma containing chyle.

25 Biliary Atresia

1) Etiology

Unknown

Inflammatory process from the prenatal period or shortly after birth

2) Pathology

An obliteration or discontinuity of the biliary ducts obstructs bile flow.

3) Clinical features

Jaundice

Acholic stool (Fig. 25-1)

Dark urine

Hepatosplenomegaly

Direct hyperbilirubinemia

Progress to hepatic fibrosis and cirrhosis

4) Diagnostic workup

Ultrasonography

- Triangular cord sign (Fig. 25-2) and small gallbladder
- Intrahepatic duct dilatation rare

Technetium-99m diisopropyl iminodiacetic acid (DISIDA) scan (Fig. 25-3)

Magnetic resonance cholangiography

Liver biopsy

Diagnostic laparoscopy or laparotomy

5) Differential diagnosis

Neonatal hepatitis, and so on

6) Surgery

Roux-en-Y hepatic portoenterostomy (Kasai operation, Fig. 25-4 and 26-4)

- As early as possible
- Usually within 8 weeks of life

Liver transplantation

- Primary (diagnosis after age 3 months?) or after failed Kasai operation
- In advanced liver failure

7) Complications

Cholangitis

Cirrhosis with portal hypertension

Liver failure

8) Prognosis

One third: successful

One third: improved, but may need liver transplantation eventually

One third: progressive and need liver transplantation

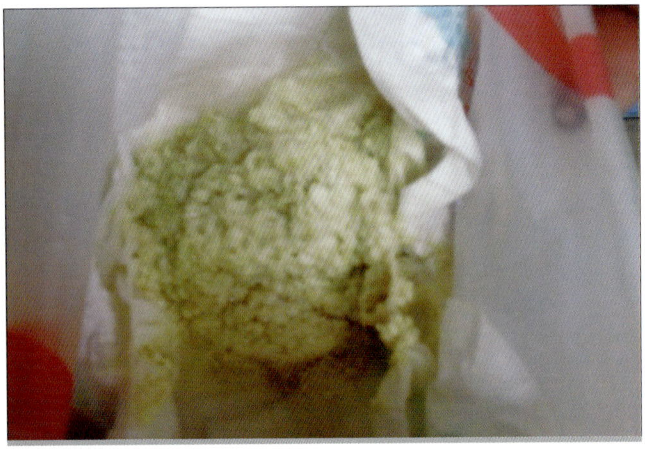

▸▸ **Fig. 25-1.** Acholic stool unmixed with bile.

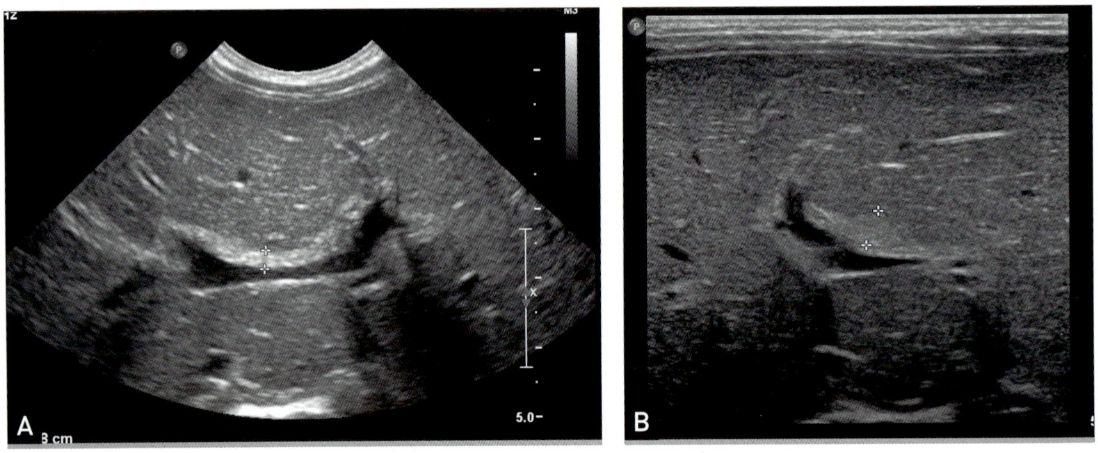

▸▸ **Fig. 25-2.** Triangular cord sign. The fibrotic remnant of the extrahepatic bile duct appears as a tubular-shaped **(A)** or triangular **(B)** density immediately cranial to the portal vein bifurcation.

Biliary Atresia

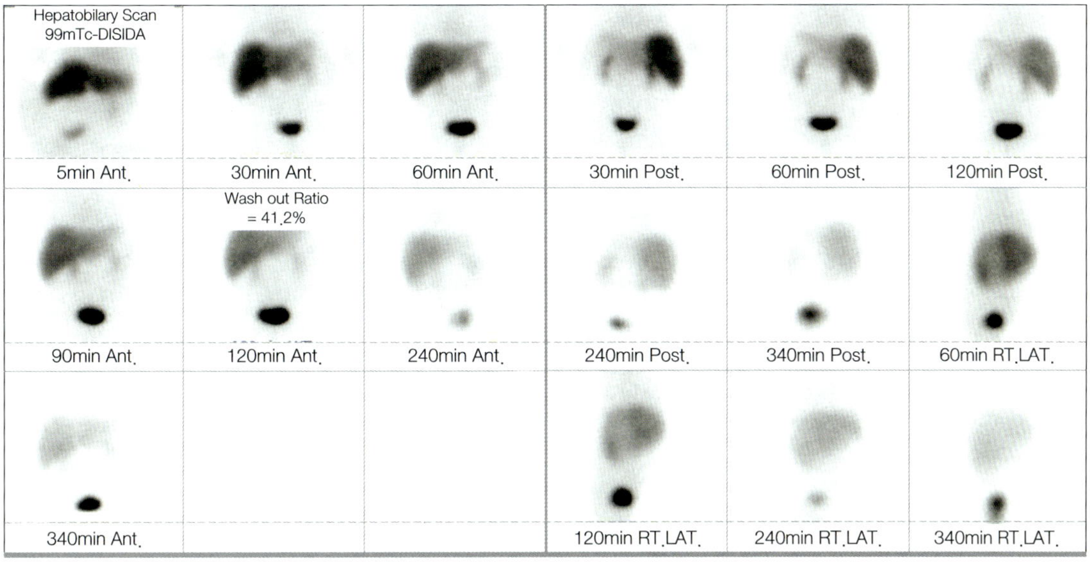

▸▸ **Fig. 25-3.** 99mTc-DISIDA scan shows no radioactivity in the intestinal tract through to 340 minutes.

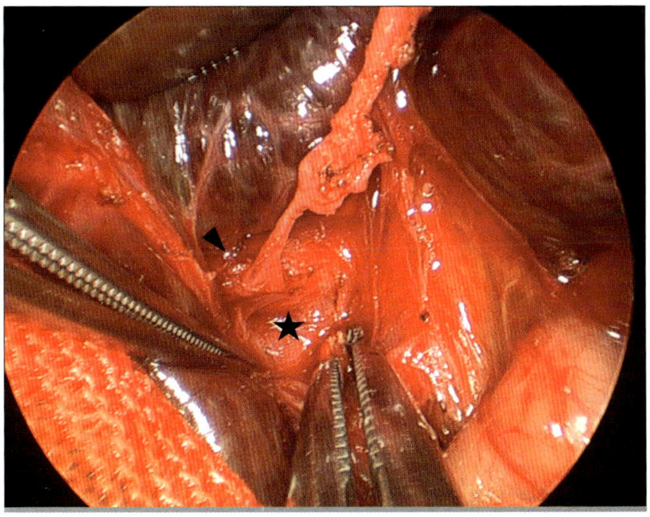

▸▸ **Fig. 25-4.** Operative findings show the atretic biliary tree and a fibrotic cord (arrowhead) cranial to the portal vein (asterisk)

26 Choledochal Cyst

1) Etiology

Many theories have been presented.

Anomalous union of the pancreatobiliary ducts: common channel theory (Fig. 26-1, 2 and 26-3)

Reflux of pancreatic enzymes into the common bile duct

2) Classification: Please refer to the articles for the schematic drawings.

Type I : cystic dilatation of the common bile duct, 85 to 95%

Type II : diverticular malformation of the common bile duct

Type III : choledochocele

Type IV : multiple cysts of the intra- or/and extrahepatic ducts

Type V : single or multiple intrahepatic cysts with normal extrahepatic duct

3) Clinical features: more common in females

Triad: abdominal pain, jaundice, mass

Cholangitis and pancreatitis

Biliary cirrhosis and malignant degeneration if untreated

4) Diagnostic workup

Ultrasonography

Computed tomography

Magnetic resonance cholangiopancreatography (Fig. 26-1 and 2)

Technetium-99m diisopropyl iminodiacetic acid (DISIDA) scan

Endoscopic retrograde cholangiopancreatography

Operative cholangiography (Fig. 26-3)

5) Differential diagnosis: so-called "correctable" type biliary atresia (Fig. 26-4)

The clinical features of infantile choledochal cyst (< 6 months of age) are very similar to those of biliary atresia.

6) Surgery

Cyst excision and Roux-en-Y hepaticojejunostomy: the standard

The anatomy should be made clear to avoid iatrogenic injuries (Fig. 26-2).

Internal drainage without cyst excision: risk of cholangitis and malignant degeneration

Unroofing of choledochocele

Segmental resection of the liver if intrahepatic duct involved

Intrahepatic duct dilatation is pathologic or secondary to distal obstruction? (Fig. 26-3)

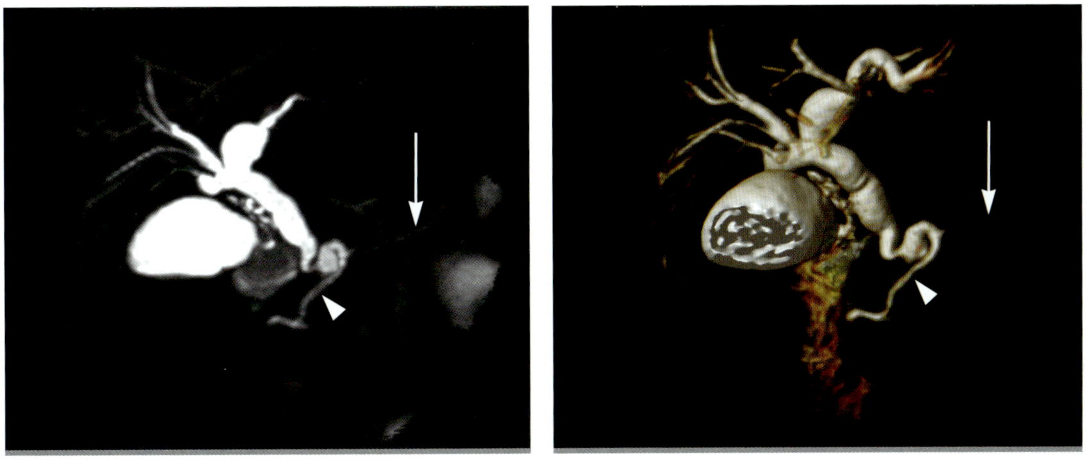

▸▸ **Fig. 26-1.** Magnetic resonance cholangiopancreatogram. The extrahepatic and proximal intrahepatic bile ducts are dilatated. The pancreatic duct (arrow) and a very long common channel (arrowhead) are demonstrated.

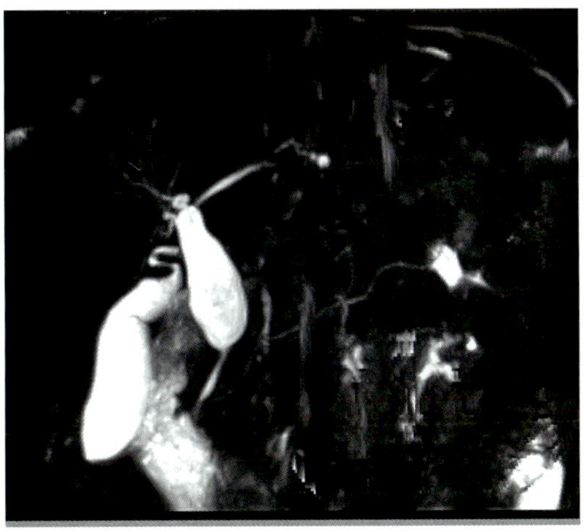

▸▸ **Fig. 26-2.** The extrahepatic bile duct shows fusiform dilatation without intrahepatic duct dilatation. The three intrahepatic ducts drain into the extrahepatic bile duct. Therefore, the anatomy of biliary and pancreatic ducts should be made clear by way of imaging studies and a view from inside the cyst to avoid iatrogenic injuries.

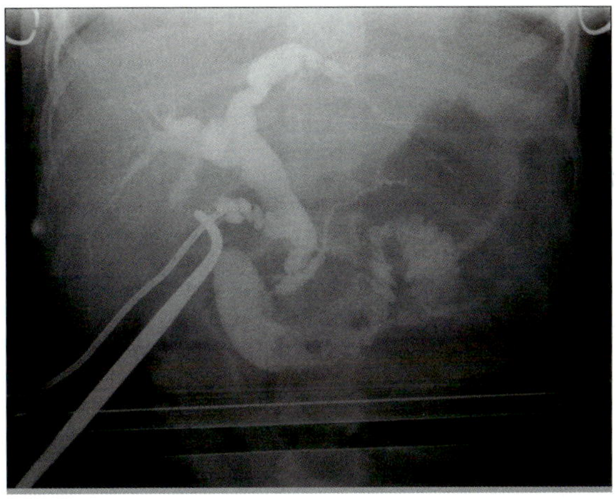

▸▸ **Fig. 26-3.** Operative cholangiogram shows dilatation of the extrahepatic and proximal intrahepatic bile ducts. The common bile duct inserts into the pancreatic duct. The dilatation of the intrahepatic ducts disappeared after surgery and was thought to be secondary to distal obstruction in this case.

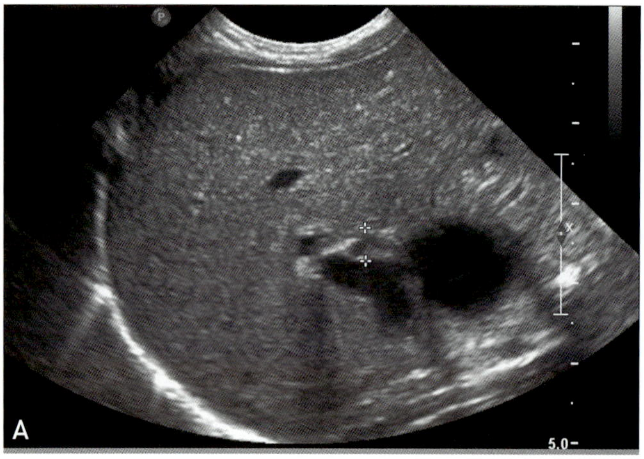

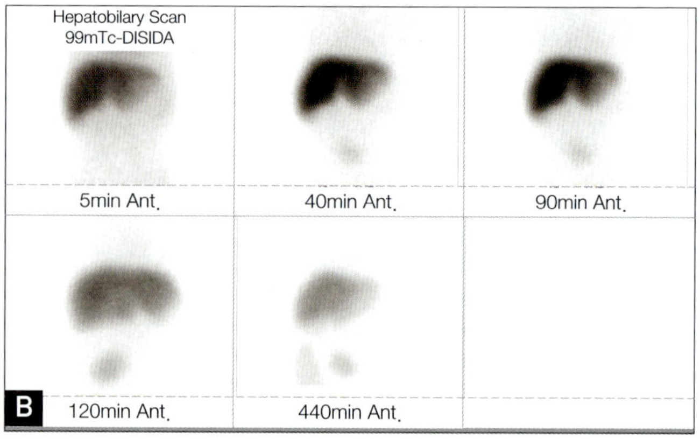

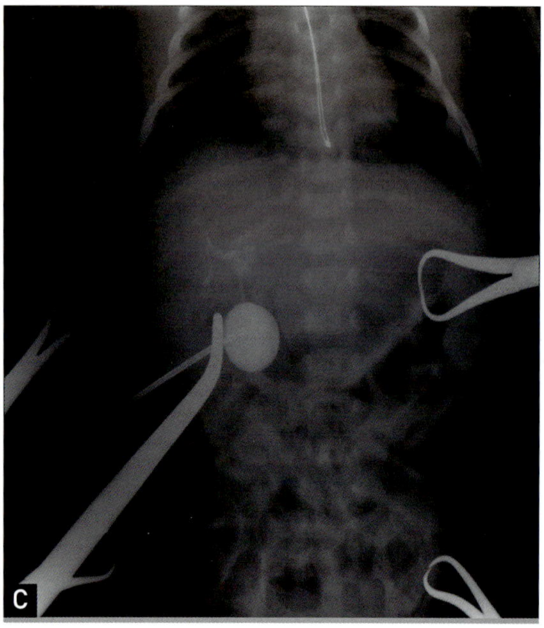

▸▸**Fig. 26-4.** Biliary atresia with a cyst, so-called correctable form. A cyst in the hepatoduodenal ligament was found with prenatal ultrasonography. **A**, Postnatal ultrasonogram shows triangular cord sign and a cyst in the hepatoduodenal ligament. **B**, DISIDA scan shows no radioactivity in the intestine. **C**, Operative cholangiogram demonstrates a biliary cyst with intrahepatic bile ducts. But, the distal duct into the duodenum is not visualized. Kasai operation is needed.

Choledochal Cyst

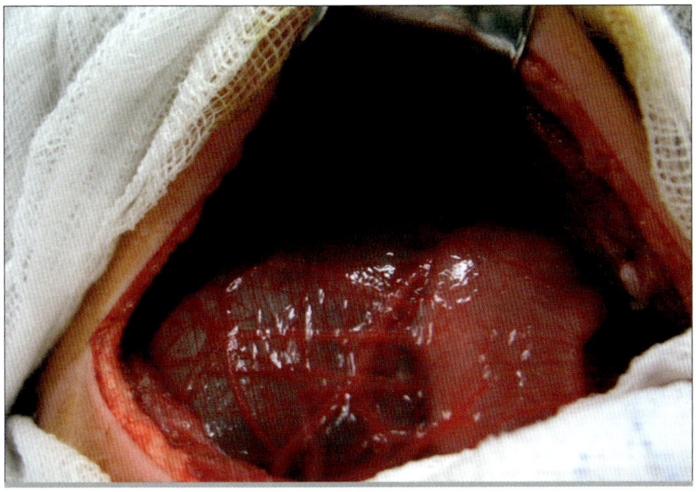

▸▸ Fig. 26-5. Operative findings showing supraduodenal cyst with vessel engorgement.

27 Inguinal hernia

1) Etiology: patent processus vaginalis (Fig. 27-1)

Processus vaginalis

A diverticulum of the peritoneum following the gonad during its descent from the retroperitoneum

Involutes in 90% of children, and leaves the tunica vaginalis

Congenital inguinal hernias are indirect hernias.

2) Incidence

Preterm > term baby

The rate of patency of the processus vaginalis is higher in the preterm.

Male > female (3 to 10 times)

The testis travels a longer way into the scrotum.

Right > left

The right testis descends later than the left.

Bilaterality is more common in girls.

3) Clinical features (Fig. 27-2 and 3)

A painless bulge in the groin or scrotum, especially during straining or crying

Reduced spontaneously when relaxed

4) Differential diagnosis

Hydrocele (Fig. 27-4)

The etiology is the same as that of inguinal hernia.

Surgery is postponed after 1 year of life because hydrocele usually resolves during the 1st year of life.

5) Incarcerated inguinal hernia

Painful irreducible mass suggests incarcerated hernia.

This can cause intestinal obstruction (Fig. 27-5).

6) Surgery (Fig. 27-6, 7 and 27-8)

High ligation of a sac: skin incision in the lowest inguinal crease

As soon as possible

Before discharge in NICU babies

The risk of incarceration is higher in the premature.

Routine contralateral exploration is not recommended.

In incarcerated hernia

Sedation, manual reduction, and elective repair after the edema subsides (24 to 48 hours later)

Emergency operation is needed in irreducible incarceration or strangulation.

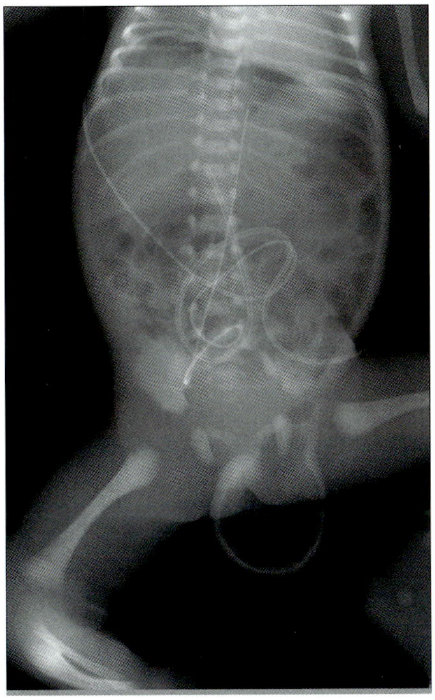

▸▸ **Fig. 27-1.** Patent processus vaginalis. The gas is shown in the scrotum through the patent processus vaginalis in a baby with pneumoperitoneum.

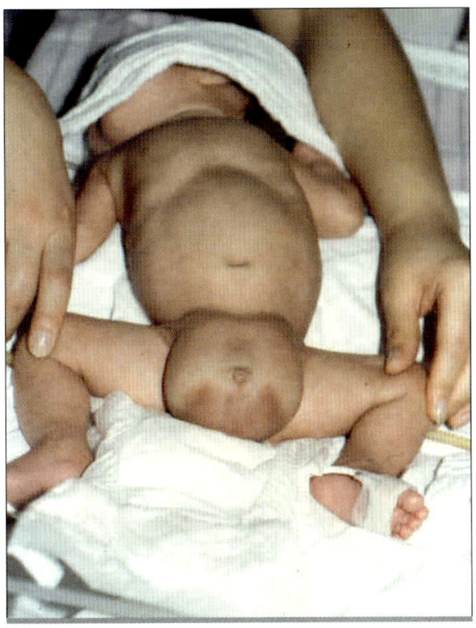

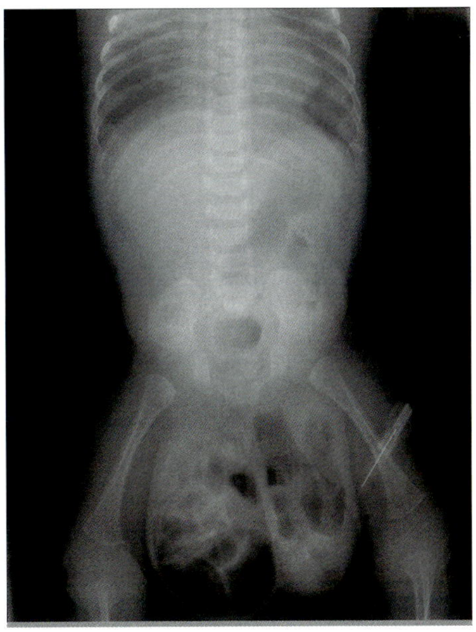

▸▸ **Fig. 27-2.** Bilateral inguinal hernia.

Inguinal hernia

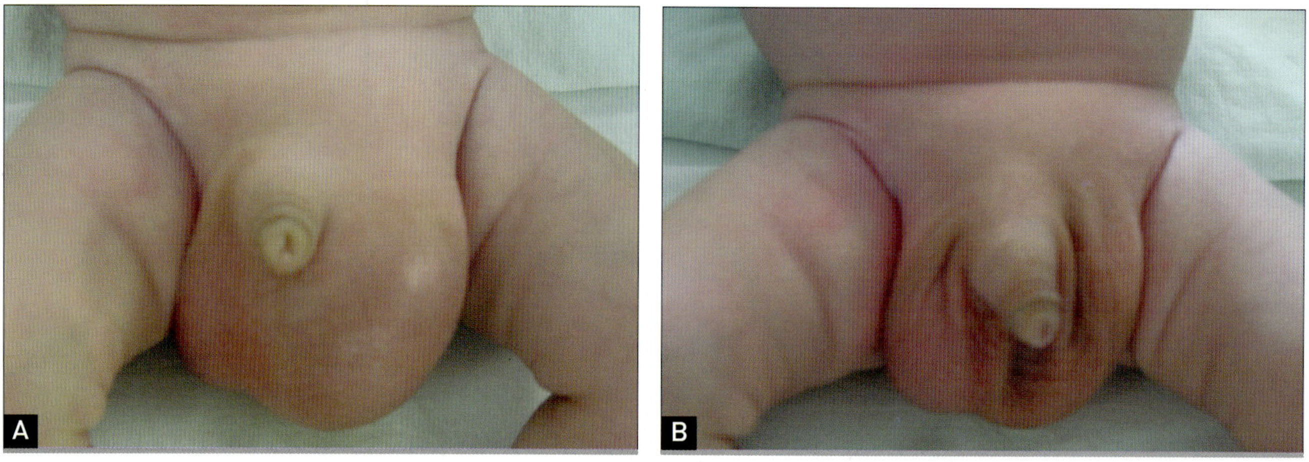

▸▸ **Fig. 27-3.** Left inguinal hernia. **A**, A bulging mass is noted in the left groin and scrotum. **B**, The mass disappears when the baby relaxes.

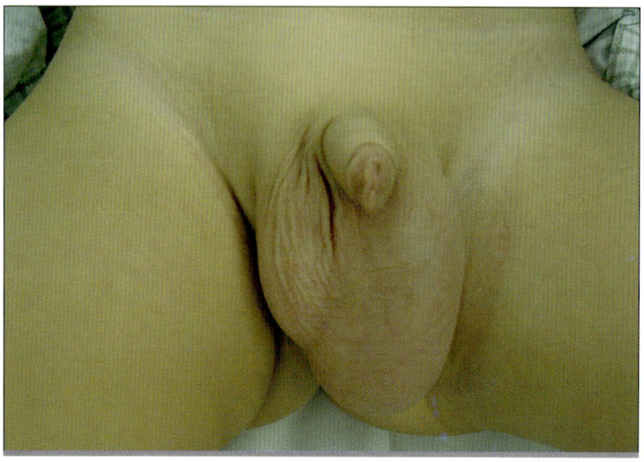

▸▸ **Fig. 27-4.** Left hydrocele. A painless, irreducible, cystic and nontender mass in the left scrotum. Note the empty groin in contrast to in inguinal hernia.

Inguinal hernia

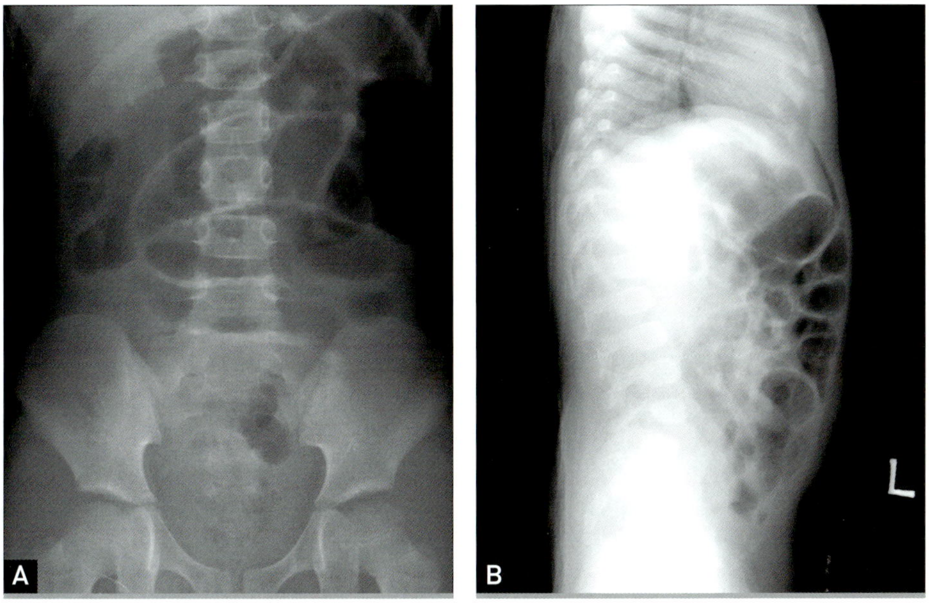

▸▸ **Fig. 27-5.** Incarcerated inguinal hernia can cause intestinal obstruction. **A**, Plain film shows dilated bowel loops. **B**, After manual reduction, cross-table lateral film shows intraperitoneal free air.

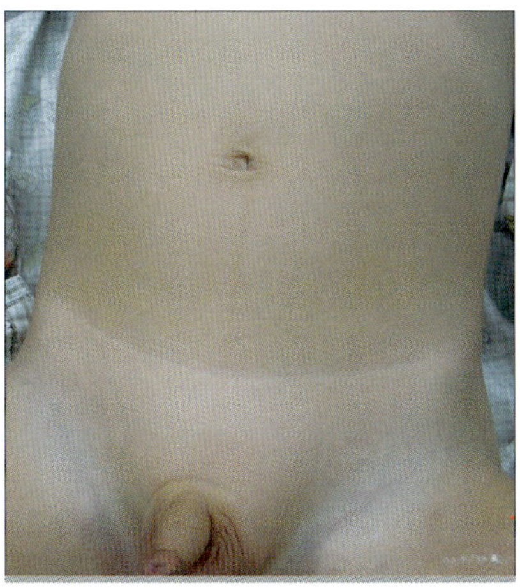

▸▸ **Fig. 27-6.** The lowest inguinal skin crease for inguinal hernia repair.

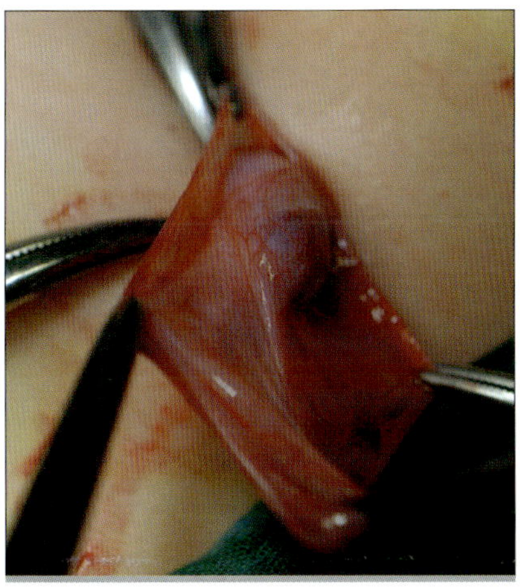

▸▸ **Fig. 27-7.** Sliding inguinal hernia in which the ovary is identified in the wall of a sac. It is recommended to place an external purse-string suture in the sac above the ovary and fallopian tube, invert the sac into the internal ring, and then close the internal ring with sutures.

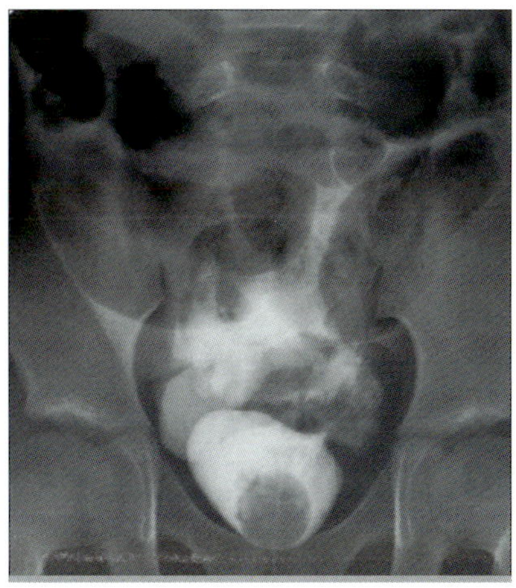

▸▸ **Fig. 27-8.** Intraperitoneal bladder rupture after mistaking the bladder as a sac during inguinal hernia repair in a girl.

28 Sacrococcygeal Teratoma

The most common congenital tumor

More common in girls

Most sacrococcygeal teratomas in newborns are benign.

Malignant transformation is possible if resection is delayed.

1) Classification

Type I : predominantly external with minimal presacral extension

Type II : primarily external with significant pelvic extension

Type III : primarily pelvic and abdominal with external extension

Type IV : entirely presacral and not visible externally

2) Clinical features

Fetal hydrops

Mass

High-output heart failure by intralesional arteriovenous shunting

Currarino triad (Chapter 22)

3) Diagnostic workup

Tumor markers: AFP, β-HCG

Plain radiography

Ultrasonography

Computed tomography

Magnetic resonance imaging

4) Surgery

Complete surgical excision including coccyx

- Posterior sacral approach: inverted chevron incision
- Abdominosacral approach

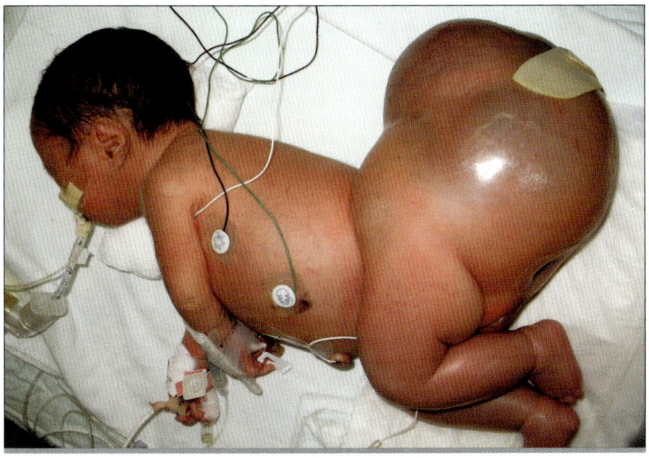

▸▸ **Fig. 28-1.** Sacrococcygeal teratoma.

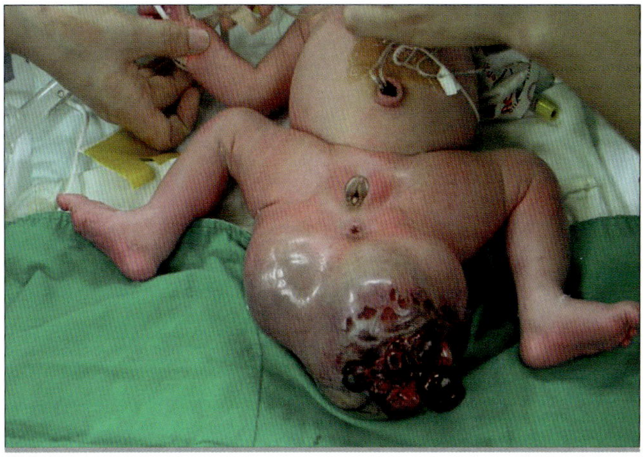

▸▸ **Fig. 28-2.** Sacrococcygeal teratoma, ruptured.

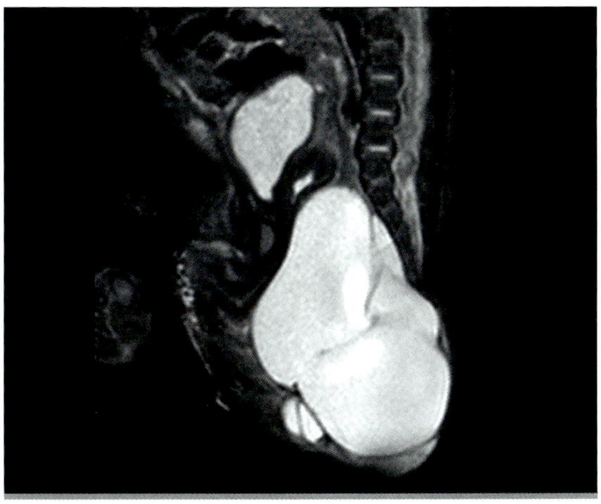

▸▸ **Fig. 28-3.** Sacrococcygeal teratoma, type III

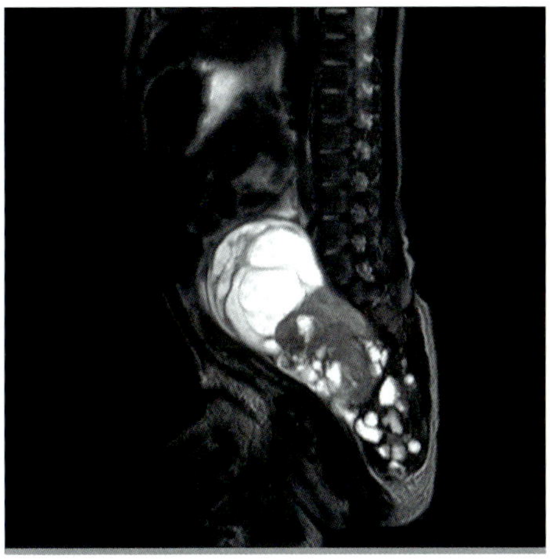

▸▸ **Fig. 28-4.** Sacrococcygeal teratoma, type IV

찾아보기

A

B

C

D

찾아보기

G

H

찾아보기

I

J

K

L

M

N

O

P

R

S

찾아보기

T

U

V

W